ECG for Nurses

ECG for Nurses

From Basics to Bedside

Archith Boloor MBBS MD (Internal Medicine)
Additional Professor and Unit Head
Department of Medicine
Kasturba Medical College, Mangalore
Manipal Academy of Higher Education
Karnataka, India

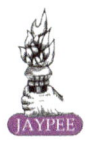

JAYPEE BROTHERS MEDICAL PUBLISHERS
The Health Sciences Publisher
New Delhi | London

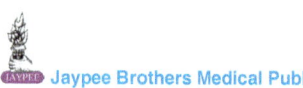
Jaypee Brothers Medical Publishers (P) Ltd

Headquarters

Jaypee Brothers Medical Publishers (P) Ltd
EMCA House
23/23-B, Ansari Road, Daryaganj
New Delhi - 110 002, India
Landline: +91-11-23272143, +91-11-23272703
+91-11-23282021, +91-11-23245672
Email: jaypee@jaypeebrothers.com

Corporate Office

Jaypee Brothers Medical Publishers (P) Ltd
4838/24, Ansari Road, Daryaganj
New Delhi 110 002, India
Phone: +91-11-43574357
Fax: +91-11-43574314
Email: jaypee@jaypeebrothers.com

Website: www.jaypeebrothers.com

Website: www.jaypeedigital.com

Overseas Office

J.P. Medical Ltd
83 Victoria Street, London
SW1H 0HW (UK)
Phone: +44 20 3170 8910
Fax: +44 (0)20 3008 6180
Email: info@jpmedpub.com

© 2024, Jaypee Brothers Medical Publishers

The views and opinions expressed in this book are solely those of the original contributor(s)/author(s) and do not necessarily represent those of editor(s) of the book.

All rights reserved. No part of this publication may be reproduced, stored or transmitted in any form or by any means, electronic, mechanical, photocopying, recording or otherwise, without the prior permission in writing of the publishers.

All brand names and product names used in this book are trade names, service marks, trademarks or registered trademarks of their respective owners. The publisher is not associated with any product or vendor mentioned in this book.

Medical knowledge and practice change constantly. This book is designed to provide accurate, authoritative information about the subject matter in question. However, readers are advised to check the most current information available on procedures included and check information from the manufacturer of each product to be administered, to verify the recommended dose, formula, method and duration of administration, adverse effects and contraindications. It is the responsibility of the practitioner to take all appropriate safety precautions. Neither the publisher nor the author(s)/editor(s) assume any liability for any injury and/or damage to persons or property arising from or related to use of material in this book.

This book is sold on the understanding that the publisher is not engaged in providing professional medical services. If such advice or services are required, the services of a competent medical professional should be sought.

Every effort has been made where necessary to contact holders of copyright to obtain permission to reproduce copyright material. If any have been inadvertently overlooked, the publisher will be pleased to make the necessary arrangements at the first opportunity.

Inquiries for bulk sales may be solicited at: jaypee@jaypeebrothers.com

ECG for Nurses

First Edition: 2024

ISBN 978-93-5696-270-5

"We should first endeavor to better understand the working of the heart in all its details, and the cause of a large variety of abnormalities. This will enable us, in a possibly still distant future and based upon a clear insight and improved knowledge, to give relief to the suffering of our patients."

—Willem Einthoven (1906)

Preface

It has been more than fifteen years now, but I still distinctly remember that night ICU duty day. I was examining a new admission patient, checking the vitals, when I heard the nurse say "Doctor, Its VT". She has just connected the ECG monitor. As I looked up, she was ready with the defibrillator, and we did resuscitate 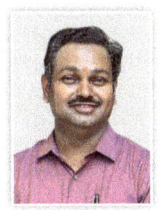 the patient quickly. There are so many instances of learning that I have acquired from the nurses and paramedics in these years. You do not need to be a doctor to read and interpret ECGs, anyone with the interest and aptitude can do it.

Reading an ECG is not necessarily the hardest thing in the world; just a couple of basic rules to follow, a few tips and tricks and a whole lot of practice. I have done the work and compiled this book with just that intention in mind—a handbook to help the primary care providers to breakdown an ECG and quickly act in emergencies.

ECGs for Nurses provides everything the nurse needs to know about the electrocardiogram. Accessible yet comprehensive, and packed with case studies, this portable guide enables nurses to become skilled practitioners in an area often seen as highly complex. Using real ECG traces as examples, possible effects on the patient and treatment options are discussed with a focus on the role of the nurse.

This fully illustrated reference guide for nurses remains the essential for working in all acute areas, as well as general nurses and students learning about ECGs for the first time.

Finally, I want you to remember that an ECG is a lot like life—if you try too hard to understand every bit of it, you will miss out on what is important. Anything out of the ordinary does not mean something is wrong, it just means you have to pay attention.

You will have your peaks, some Himalayan, some not. You will have your dips, sometimes longer than usual. Learn to appreciate them.

Because without those highs and lows, you will have a flat line.

Archith Boloor
archithb@gmail.com

Contributers

Mohammed Shaheen
Resident
Department of Emergency Medicine
Hamad Medical Corporation
Doha, Qatar

Mohamed Faizan Thouseef
Senior Resident
Department of Internal Medicine
Kasturba Medical College, Mangalore
Manipal Academy of Higher Education
Karnataka, India

Ashwini MV
Senior Resident
Department of Cardiology
Kasturba Medical College, Mangalore
Manipal Academy of Higher Education
Karnataka, India

GG Akshay Prabhu
Resident
Department of Internal Medicine
Kasturba Medical College, Mangalore
Manipal Academy of Higher Education
Karnataka, India

T Chyavan Trisule Reddy

Resident
Department of Internal Medicine
Kasturba Medical College, Mangalore
Manipal Academy of Higher Education
Karnataka, India

Murali Mohan R

Department of Internal Medicine
Kasturba Medical College, Mangalore
Manipal Academy of Higher Education
Karnataka, India

Acknowledgments

It is now over a century (127 years, actually) since Willem Einthoven invented the first practical electrocardiograph to register the electrical activity of the human heart. Since then, the ECG has become part of routine workup in clinical practice and is used for the diagnosis and management of a variety of cardiac and non-cardiac disorders. Even a century after the discovery of the ECG, newer ECG patterns are being discovered.

This handbook is not designed as a classic textbook that covers all aspects of the subject, nor is it meant to discuss other cellular and imaging modalities related to this topic. I have attempted to make this handbook easy to use and understand; therefore, I believe it should be in the hands of any first care response person who read ECGs as their very own.

My sincere thanks to Dr Mohammed Shaheen, Dr Ashwini MV, Dr GG Akshay Prabhu, Dr Mohamed Faizan Thouseef, Dr T Chyavan Trisule Reddy, and Dr Murali Mohan R, for their contribution to this book.

I thank Dr Sheetal Raj M, Dr Anudeep Padakanti, Dr Vivek K Koushik, Dr Abu Thajudeen, Dr Madhav Hande, and Dr Nikhil Kenny Thomas, for their presence in my life—a source of constant inspiration, encouragement, and joy.

I thank my family and my friends, both in and out of the medical fraternity, who have played their irreplaceable role in bringing me to where we are today.

I convey my sincere thanks to Shri Jitendar P Vij (Group Chairman), Mr Ankit Vij (Managing Director), and Mr MS Mani (Group President) of M/s Jaypee Brothers Medical Publishers (P) Ltd, New Delhi, India, for having been the guiding force behind all my works.

I also thank Dr Madhu Choudhary (Director-Educational Publishing), Ms Pooja Bhandari [Director-Production

(Books and Journals)], Ms Sunita Katla (Executive Assistant to Group Chairman and Publishing Manager), Ms Samina Khan (Executive Assistant to Publishing Head-Education), Dr Aditya Tayal (Team Lead-UG Publishing), Ms Alisha Talwar (Content Strategist), Mr Rajesh Sharma (Production Coordinator), Ms Seema Dogra (Cover Visualizer), Ms Neelam Kakriya (Proofreader), Mr Kapil Dev Sharma (Typesetter), and Mr Gopal Singh Kirola (Graphic Designer) of M/s Jaypee Brothers Medical Publishers (P) Ltd, New Delhi, India, for their help in the formatting and their well-received technical assistance and unwavering support during the process of developing this project.

This book has been written considering the need of Nurses as the first response persons in the emergency team. I welcome any and every feedback, and I assure you that I will strive to improve this book and keep it up to date for further editions.

Lastly, I thank Mother Goddess for what was, what is, and what will be.

Contents

1. **Introduction, Anatomical and Physiological Consideration**   1
   - ❖ **The Cardiac Conduction System: *The Wiring System of the Heart* 1**
     - Origin and Spread of Cardiac Excitation 2
     - Impulse Conduction through the Heart 3
     - SA Node of Keith and Flack 4
     - Internodal Conduction Pathways 4
     - The AV Node 5
     - The Bundle of His and the Bundle Branches 5
     - Purkinje Fibers or Purkinje Cardiomyocytes 6
   - ❖ **ECG Waveforms 6**
     - J Wave and U Wave 7

2. **Technical Aspects of ECG**   10
     - What is an ECG? 10
     - Utility of ECG: With ECGs We Can Identify 11
   - ❖ **ECG Paper and Timing 11**
     - ECG Leads 13
     - Placement of Electrodes 15
     - Standard Sites Unavailable 15
     - Precordial Leads 18
     - Color Codes Given by AHA 18
     - Limb Leads Electrodes 20
     - Ambulatory ECG Monitoring 27
   - ❖ **Procedure of Obtaining an ECG: A Step by Step Checklist 30**
     - Electrode Placement 31
     - Limb Electrode and Lead Placement 34
     - Recording the ECG Trace 35
     - Completion of Procedure 36

3. Rate, Rhythm, and Axis   37

- ❖ **Reading 12-Lead ECG** 37
- ❖ **Rate** 37
  - Rule of 300 37
  - 6-Second Rule 39
  - For Irregular Rhythms 39
- ❖ **Rhythm 40**
  - Determine Regularity 40
  - Normal Sinus Rhythm—P Wave followed by QRS 41
  - Sinus Bradycardia 41
  - Sinus Tachycardia 42
  - Sinus Pause 42
  - Atrial Fibrillation 42
  - Atrial Flutter 43
  - Ventricular Fibrillation 43
  - Ventricular Tachycardia 43
  - Torsades de Pointes 44
  - Supraventricular Tachycardia 44
- ❖ **Axis 44**
  - The QRS Axis 44
  - Cardiac Axis 45
  - Determining the Axis 45
- ❖ **Cardiac Axis Thumb Rule 49**

4. Waves, Segments, and Intervals   51

- ❖ **Understanding ECG Waveform** 51
- ❖ **P Waves 52**
  - Assess the P waves 52
  - Abnormalities of P Wave 52
  - Other P Wave Abnormalities 54
- ❖ **PR Interval 54**
  - Atrioventricular Block 55
  - Short PR Interval 57
- ❖ **PR Segment 57**
- ❖ **QRS Complex 58**
- ❖ **Low Voltage QRS 60**
- ❖ **High Voltage QRS Complexes 61**
  - Bundle Branch Blocks 63
- ❖ **J Point 66**

- ❖ ST Segment 66
- ❖ T Wave 68
- ❖ QT-Interval 75
- ❖ U Wave 77

5. ECG in Myocardial Infarction 78
- ❖ **Acute Coronary Syndrome 78**
- ❖ **Myocardial Infarction 78**
  - ECG Changes: Ischemia 79
  - ECG Changes: Injury 79
  - ECG Changes: Infarct 82
  - Evolving MI and Hallmarks of AMI 82
  - Reciprocal Changes 82
- ❖ **Localization of MI Based on ECG 82**
- ❖ **Non-ST Elevation Myocardial Infarction 85**
  - ECG manifestation 85
- ❖ **Complications of Acute Coronary Syndrome 86**

6. Tachyarrhythmia 88
  - Narrow QRS Complex 89
  - Wide QRS Complex 89
- ❖ **Narrow Complex Tachydysrhythmias 89**
  - Sinus Rhythm 89
  - Sinus Tachycardia 90
  - Atrial Flutter 91
  - Supraventricular Tachycardia 93
  - Atrial Fibrillation 95
  - Premature Ventricular Complex 97
  - Idioventricular Rhythm 99
  - Ventricular Tachycardia (VT) 101
  - Torsades de Pointes 104
  - Ventricular Fibrillation 105

7. Bradyarrhythmias 107
- ❖ **Sinus Bradycardia 107**
  - ECG Characteristics 107
  - Causes 107
  - Medical Management 107
- ❖ **Heart Block 108**
  - AV Block 108

- Sinus Node Dysfunction (SND)/Sick Sinus Syndrome 111

8. Electrolytes and ECG 113
- ❖ **Potassium Disorders 113**
  - ECG Features of Hyperkalemia 113
  - ECG Features of Hypokalemia 117
- ❖ **Calcium Disorders 118**
  - ECG Features of Hypocalcemia 118
  - ECG Features of Hypercalcemia 118

9. Drugs and Miscellaneous 120
- ❖ **Digoxin Effect 120**
- **Miscellaneous 121**
- ❖ **Pericarditis 121**
- ❖ **Pulmonary Embolism 121**
- ❖ **Pacing in ECG 123**
  - Atrial Pacing 123
  - Ventricular Pacing 123
  - Atrial and Ventricular Pacing 124

10. Review—Multiple Choice Questions 125

11. Practice ECGs 145

Appendices 183

Index 187

Terminology

- **Electrocardiogram (ECG)**: A test that measures the electrical activity of the heart.
- **P wave**: The first deflection in an ECG waveform that represents the electrical activity of the atria.
- **QRS complex**: This refers to the three waves that follow the P wave and represent the electrical activity of the ventricles.
- **T wave**: The final wave in an ECG waveform that represents the ventricular repolarization.
- **ST segment**: The section of the ECG waveform that connects the QRS complex and the T wave and represents the time between ventricular depolarization and repolarization.
- **PR interval**: This refers to the time from the start of the P wave to the start of the QRS complex and represents the time it takes for an electrical impulse to travel from the atria to the ventricles.
- **QT interval**: This is the time between the start of the Q wave and the end of the T wave and represents the total time it takes for ventricular depolarization and repolarization.
- **Arrhythmia**: A condition where the heart beats irregularly, either too fast or too slow.
- **Artifact**: A disturbance in the ECG signal that may be caused by movement, muscle activity, or electrical interference.
- **Bradycardia**: A heart rate that is slower than normal.
- **Tachycardia**: A heart rate that is faster than normal.
- **Atrial fibrillation:** A type of arrhythmia where the atria of the heartbeat irregularly.
- **Sinus rhythm**: A normal heart rhythm where the electrical activity of the heart originates from the sinus node.

Introduction, Anatomical and Physiological Consideration

CHAPTER 1

THE CARDIAC CONDUCTION SYSTEM: *THE WIRING SYSTEM OF THE HEART*

The human heart beats 2.5 billion times during a normal lifespan, a feat accomplished by cells of the cardiac conduction system (CCS). The functional components of the CCS can be broadly divided into the impulse generating nodes and the impulse propagating His-Purkinje system.

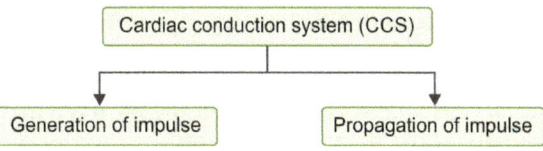

- ❖ The heart is controlled by the autonomic nervous system (predominantly by vagus nerve's parasympathetic branch). It increases/decreases contraction, but it does not initiate it.
- ❖ The heart has its own regulating system known as the conduction system.
- ❖ The conduction system is composed of specialized muscle tissue that generates action potentials within the cardiac tissue.
- ❖ The conduction system of the heart consists of the following **(Fig. 1):**
  - ◆ Sinoatrial (SA) node (pacemaker of the heart)
  - ◆ Atrioventricular (AV) node
  - ◆ Internodal atrial pathway
  - ◆ Bundle of His and bundle branches
    - Right
    - Left
      » Anterior fascicle
      » Posterior fascicle
  - ◆ Purkinje system

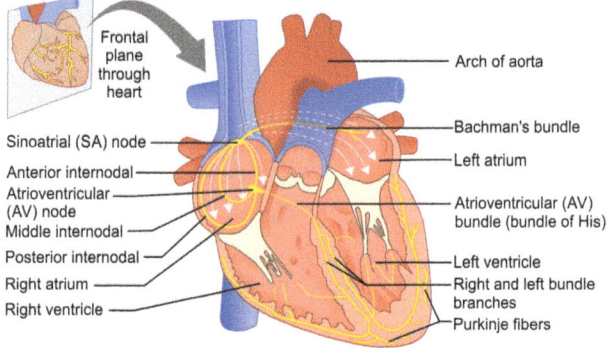

Fig. 1: Conduction system of the heart.

Origin and Spread of Cardiac Excitation

- The rate and rhythm of the heart are controlled by the SA node situated at the junction of superior vena cava (SVC) and right atrium
- The impulse from the SA node spreads through the atrial musculature and down to the AV node that is situated above the tricuspid valve.
- Passage through the AV node is relatively slow, accounting for the normal physiological delay in ventricular depolarization. This delay prevents the contraction of atria and ventricles at the same time.
- The impulse then travels downward to the bundle of His and through its branches (right bundle branch and left bundle branch) to the Purkinje network of fibers that convey the impulse to the ventricular endocardium and then epicardium.
- The last part of the heart to be depolarized are the *posterobasal portion of the left ventricle (LV), the pulmonary conus, and the upper most portion of the septum.*
- The SA node is the normal pacemaker of the heart as it has the fastest inherent discharge rate. However, potential pace making properties also exist in the cells of the AV node, bundle of His, and Purkinje fibers.
- The SA node is the dominant pacemaker with an intrinsic rate of 60–100 beats/minute.

Chapter 1: Introduction, Anatomical and Physiological...

- AV node: Back-up pacemaker with an intrinsic rate of 40–60 beats/minute.
- Ventricular cells: Back-up pacemaker with an intrinsic rate of 20–45 beats/minute.

Impulse Conduction through the Heart

The impulse conduction through heart has been explained in **Figure 2**.

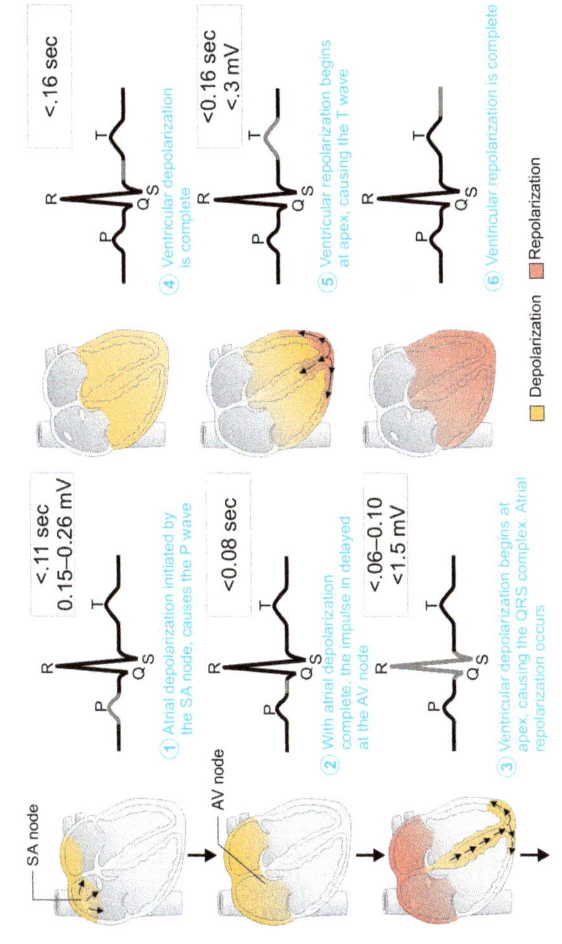

Fig. 2: Impulse conduction through heart.

① Atrial depolarization initiated by the SA node, causes the P wave (<.11 sec, 0.15–0.26 mV)

② With atrial depolarization complete, the impulse in delayed at the AV node (<0.08 sec)

③ Ventricular depolarization begins at apex, causing the QRS complex. Atrial repolarization occurs (<.06–0.10, <1.5 mV)

④ Ventricular depolarization is complete (<.16 sec)

⑤ Ventricular repolarization begins at apex, causing the T wave (<0.16 sec, <.3 mV)

⑥ Ventricular repolarization is complete

Table 1: Rates of conduction of impulses.

Tissue	Conduction rate (m/s)	Relative value
SA node	0.05	Second least
Atrial pathway	1	
AV node	0.02–0.05	Least
Bundle of His	1	
Purkinje system	4	Highest
Ventricular muscle	1	

Purkinje system is the fastest and AV node is the slowest.

The rates of conduction of impulses through the various tissues in the conduction system of the heart are shown in **Table 1.**

SA Node of Keith and Flack

- SA node is the pacemaker of the heart.
- It lies at junction of right atrial appendage with the SVC.
- It underlies the uppermost part of sulcus terminalis.
- SA node has the highest intrinsic rate of impulse generation.
- Dimensions of SA node: 10–20 mm length × 1 mm thickness × 3 mm wide.
- Composition of SA node: Specialized branching myocardial fibers embedded in dense matrix of fibrous tissue.
  - The P-cells are normal impulse forming cells
  - The T-cells are located at the margins of the sinus node with the atrial myocardium and they help in the distribution of impulses formed in the P-cells to the atrial myocardium
- Artery to SA node: 55%—right coronary artery (RCA), 5%—circumflex branch of left coronary artery (LCA)

Why SA node leads the heart?

SAN leads the heart as it has the highest rate of impulse generation. Rate of impulse generation is shown in **Table 2.**

Internodal Conduction Pathways

- These are the special pathways in atrial wall.
- Histologically, they are a mixture of Purkinje fiber and ordinary cardiac muscle cells.

Table 2: Rate of impulse generation of various tissues.	
Tissue	**Rate of impulse generation**
SA node	70–80/min
AV node	40–60/min
Bundle of His	40/min
Purkinje system	24/min

- These pathways function to transmit impulses rapidly from SA node to AV node
- There are three internodal pathways, namely:
  1. Anterior internodal tract of Bachman-James
  2. Middle internodal tract of Wenckebach
  3. Posterior internodal tract of Thoral
- Accessory pathway: Via these pathways, impulse can directly travel to the ventricles.

The AV Node

- AV node is the pathway through which sinus impulse can reach ventricles.
- Also known as the node of Tawara
- It lies subendocardially in medial wall of right atrium
- Artery to AV node: 90%—RCA, 10%—circumflex branch of LCA
- AV node dealy: AV node slow down the sinus impulse so that both atria and ventricle do not contract at same.

The Bundle of His and the Bundle Branches

- The AV node continues as bundle of His which is a short structure bifurcates into right and left bundles.
- The right bundle is the direct continuation of the His bundle. Hence, the impulse first goes to the right bundle branch, then to the left bundle branch
- The left bundle divides into anterosuperior and posteroinferior fascicles **(Fig. 3)**
- Blood supply: The His bundle gets blood supply from both left anterior descending (LAD) and posterior descending artery. Blood supply of the bundle branches is from septal branches of LAD and AV nodal branch of RCA.

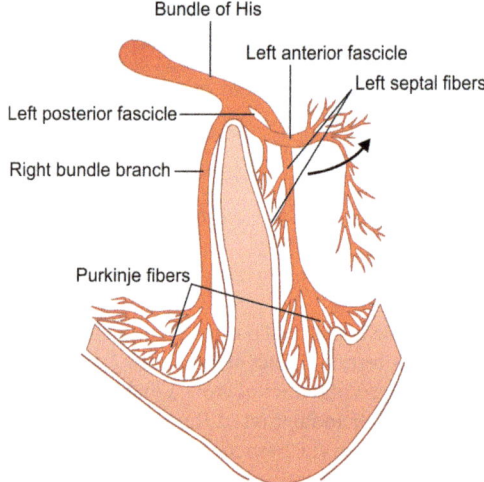

Fig. 3: Bundle branches and Purkinje fibers.

Purkinje Fibers or Purkinje Cardiomyocytes

It forms terminal part of conducting system. Purkinje fibers play an important role in cardiac conduction and arrhythmogenesis. Purkinje cell action potentials are longer than their ventricular counterpart, and display two levels of resting potential. Purkinje cells provide for rapid propagation of the cardiac impulse to ventricular cells and have pacemaker and triggered activity, which differs from ventricular cells.

ECG WAVEFORMS

- **P wave**: Denotes atrial depolarization
- **QRS complex**: Denotes depolarization of ventricles
  - If the initial QRS depletion in a particular lead is negative, it is termed a Q wave
  - The first positive deflection is termed an R wave.
  - A negative deflection after an R wave is an S wave.
  - Subsequent positive or negative waves are labeled "R" and "S", respectively

- Lowercase letters (qrs) are used for waves of relatively small amplitude
- An entirely negative QRS complex is termed a QS wave.

❖ **T waves**: Denotes the repolarization (or recovery) of the ventricles.
- The interval from the beginning of the QRS complex to the apex of the T wave is referred to as the absolute refractory period.
- The last half of the T wave is referred to as the relative refractory period

❖ **PR interval**: It is from the beginning of the P wave to the beginning of the QRS-complex. Includes atrial depolarization + delay in the AV junction. This delay allows time for the atria to contract before the ventricles contract.

Note: Atrial repolarization is usually too low in amplitude to be detected, but it may become apparent in conditions, such as acute pericarditis and atrial infarction.

❖ **ST segment**: ST segment is isoelectric and at the same level as subsequent PR interval. It is the length between the end of the S wave (end of ventricular depolarization) and the beginning of repolarization. It is measured from the J point on the end of QRS complex, to inclination of T wave.

❖ **QT interval**: Is from the beginning of the QRS complex to the end of T wave.

The QT interval incudes both ventricular depolarization and repolarization and varies inversely with the heart rate. A rate-related QT interval, QTc ("Corrected" Bazzet's formula is QT/Square root of RR interval), can be calculated and is normally 0.44 seconds (Some references give QTc upper normal limit as 0.43 seconds in men and 0.45 seconds in women) **(Fig. 4)**.

What differentiates a segment from an interval?

A segment is a straight line connecting two waves. An interval encompasses at least one wave plus the connecting straight line.

J Wave and U Wave

J point: J point is the point at which the QRS complex meets the ST segment. It is an isoelectric point and its importance lies in the fact that ST segment elevation is measured with respect to it.

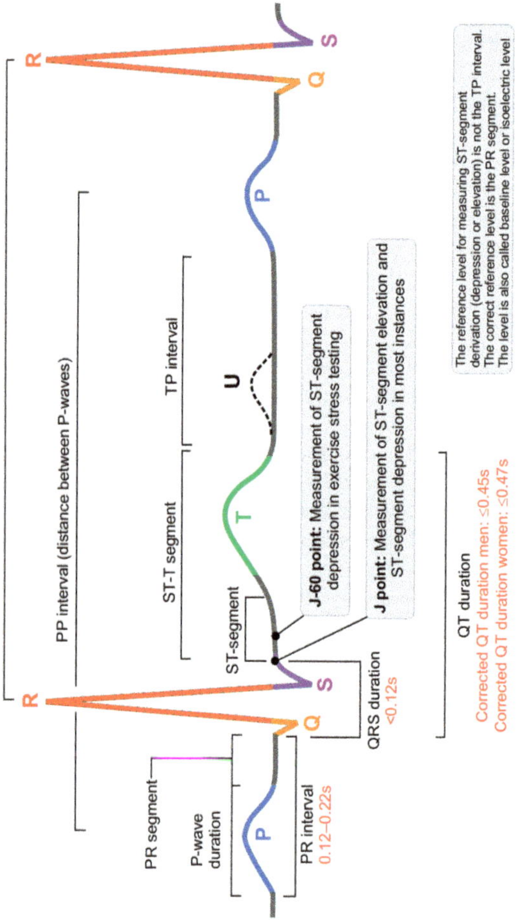

Chapter 1: Introduction, Anatomical and Physiological...

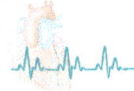

Fig. 4: ECG waveforms.

J wave: J wave is a positive deflection occurring at the junction between the QRS complex and ST segment (J point) observed in people suffering from hypothermia with a temperature <32°C (**Fig. 5**).

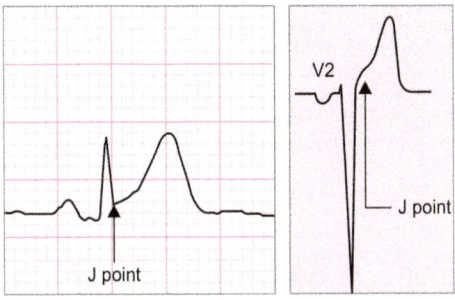

Fig. 5: J wave.

U wave: U waves are thought to represent repolarization of the papillary muscles or Purkinje fibers. Typically small, and by definition, follows the T wave. Prominent U waves are most often seen in hypokalemia, but may be present in hypercalcemia, thyrotoxicosis.

Technical Aspects of ECG

CHAPTER 2

INTRODUCTION

What is an ECG?

- The electrocardiogram (ECG) is a representation of the electrical events of the cardiac cycle.
- Each event has a distinctive waveform. The electrical impulses can be recorded by placing electrodes to the different areas of the body.
- Thus, if a left arm electrode is connected to the positive pole of a galvanometer and a right arm electrode is connected to the negative pole, the magnitude as well as the direction of the electrical impulse can be measured.
- The height of the ECG deflection represents the difference in potential between the two electrodes.
- The first ECG from the intact human heart was recorded with a mercury capillary electrometer by Augustus Waller in May 1887 at St. Mary's Hospital, London. The tracings were poor and exhibited only two distorted deflections (**Fig. 1**).
- Willem Einthoven (1860-1927) who was professor of physiology at the University of Leiden, The Netherlands, began his studies of the ECG with the mercury capillary electrometer, and improved its distortion mathematically, so that he was finally able to register a good representation of

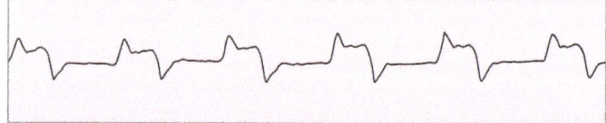

Fig. 1: The first ECG from intact human heart.

the ECG before the beginning of the twentieth century. Later, he further improved ECG recordings with the introduction of a string galvanometer of his design.

- Einthoven developed a system of electrocardiographic standardization that continues to be used all over the world and introduced the triaxial bipolar system with three limb leads and thus established uniformity of the recording process. Einthoven also conceived the famous equilateral triangle with leads I, II, and III at its sides and the calculation of the electrical axis (in the frontal plane) depicted as a single vector with an arrow at the center of the triangle. He was awarded the Nobel Prize in 1924 in physiology and medicine, "for the discovery of the mechanism of the ECG" **(Fig. 2)**.
- Several advances have occurred since then and the conventional 12 lead ECG records the difference in potential between electrodes placed on the surface of the body.

Utility of ECG: With ECGs We Can Identify

- Chamber hypertrophy
- Arrhythmias
- Ischemic heart disease (IHD)
- Pericarditis
- Electrolyte disturbances
- Drug toxicity

ECG PAPER AND TIMING

- ECG paper speed = 25 mm/sec
- Standardization of ECG amplitude scale **(Fig. 3)**
- Voltage calibration 1 mV = 1 cm
- Standard calibrations of the ECG paper **(Fig. 4)**:
  - Each small square = 1 mm
  - Each large square = 5 mm
- Timings:
  - 1 small square = 0.04 sec
  - 1 large square = 0.2 sec
  - 25 small squares = 1 sec
  - 5 large squares = 1 sec

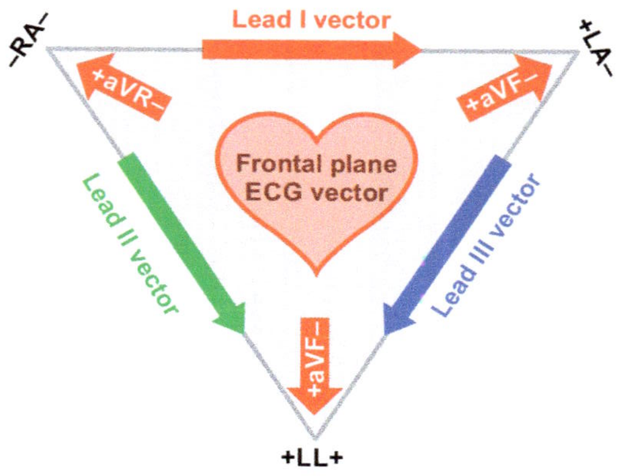

Chapter 2: Technical Aspects of ECG

Einthoven's triangle is an imaginary formation of three limb leads in a triangle used in electrocardiography, formed by the two shoulders and the pubis. The shape forms an inverted equilateral triangle with the heart at the center that produces zero potential when the voltages are summed. It is named after Willem Einthoven, who theorized its existence. Einthoven used these measuring points, by immersing the hands and foot in pails of salt water, as the contacts for his string galvanometer, the first practical ECG machine

Lead placements:

Lead I: This axis goes from shoulder to shoulder with the negative electrode placed on the right shoulder and the positive electrode placed on the left shoulder. This results in a 0° angle of orientation

I = LA − RA (I = LA − RA)

Lead II: This axis goes from the right arm to the left leg, with the negative electrode on the shoulder and the positive one on the leg. This results in a +60° angle of orientation

II = LL − RA (II = LL − RA)

Lead III: This axis goes from the left shoulder (negative electrode) to the right or left leg (positive electrode). This results in a +120° angle of orientation

III = LL − LA (III = LL − LA)

Fig. 2: Einthoven equilateral triangle.

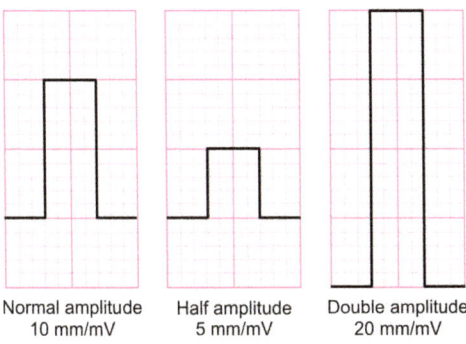

Fig. 3: ECG amplitude scale.

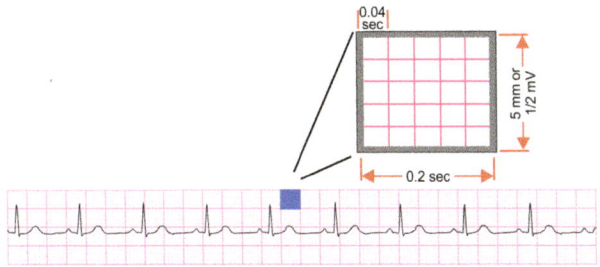

Fig. 4: Standard calibrations of the ECG paper.

ECG Leads

- An ECG is a recording of the electrical activity of the heart
- Different "views" of the heart can be recorded using different electrodes
- Electrodes are able to measure the voltages of the cardiac current
- Electrodes should be selected for maximum adhesiveness and minimum discomfort, electrical noise, and skin-electrode impedance
- Effective contact between electrode and skin is essential **(Fig. 5)**

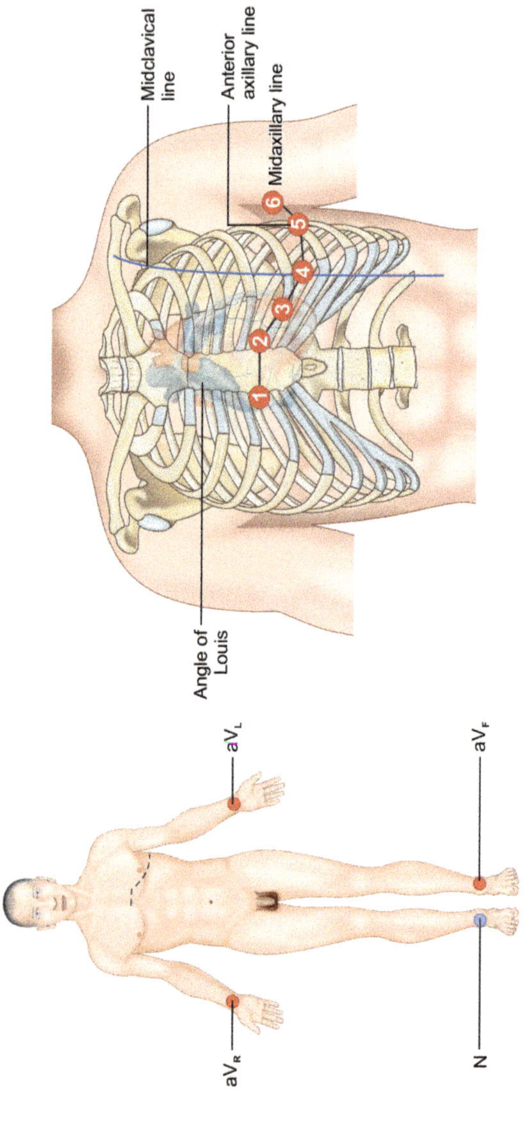

Chapter 2: Technical Aspects of ECG

Fig. 5: ECG leads.

- The standard ECG consists of 12 leads:
  - Three bipolar limb leads (I, II, and III): Oriented in the coronal plane
  - Three augmented limb leads (aVR, aVL, and aVF): Oriented in the coronal plane
  - Six unipolar precordial leads (V1–V6): Oriented in horizontal plane

Placement of Electrodes

- V1: Fourth intercostal space to the right of the sternum.
- V2: Fourth intercostal space to the left of the sternum.
- V3: Directly between leads V2 and V4.
- V4: Fifth intercostal space at the left midclavicular line.
- V5: Level with V4 at left anterior axillary line.
- V6: Level with V5 at left midaxillary line.

Standard Sites Unavailable

Patient pathology: Amputation or burns or bandages: Leads should be placed as closely as possible to the standard sites.

Specific Cardiac Abnormalities and Alternate Lead Placements

- Sinus inversus dextrocardia: Right and left arm electrodes should be reversed and precordial leads should be recorded from V1R (V2) to V6
- RVH and RV infarction: Obtain V3R and V4R
  - V4R, which is obtained by placing the V4 electrode in the 5th right intercostal space in the midclavicular line.
  - ST elevation in V4R has a sensitivity of 88%, specificity of 78%, and diagnostic accuracy of 83% in the diagnosis of RV MI.

V7, V8, and V9: V_7 is located at the left posterior axillary line at the same level as V6. V8 is located just below the angle of the left scapula at the same level as V7 and V9 just lateral to the spine at the same level as V8. These leads supplement the 12-lead ECG in the diagnosis of posterolateral ST elevation MI and should be recorded when reciprocal ST segment depression is present in V1 to V3 (**Fig. 6**).

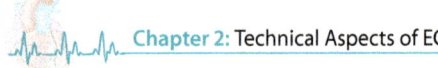

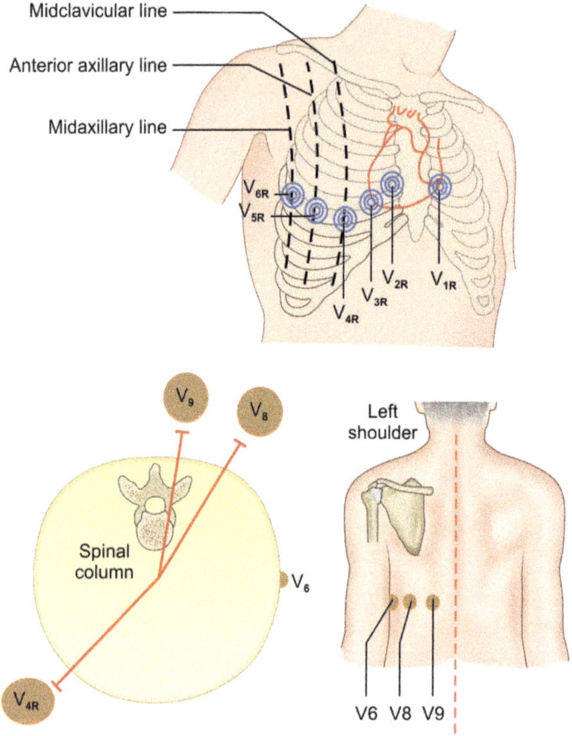

Fig. 6: Lead placement in special situations.

Formation of waveforms:
- A positive (upright) deflection is recorded in a lead, if a wave of depolarization spreads toward the positive pole of the lead
- A negative deflection is recorded, if the wave spreads toward the negative pole
- If the orientation of the depolarization vector is at right angles to a particular lead axis, then a biphasic (equally positive and negative) deflection will be recorded **(Figs. 7 to 10)**.

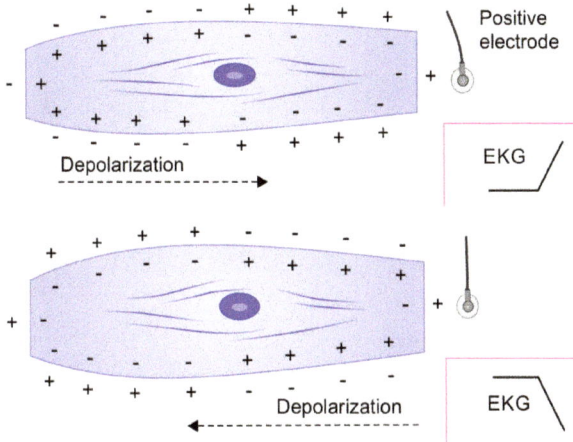

Fig. 7: Formation of waves—positive and negative deflection.

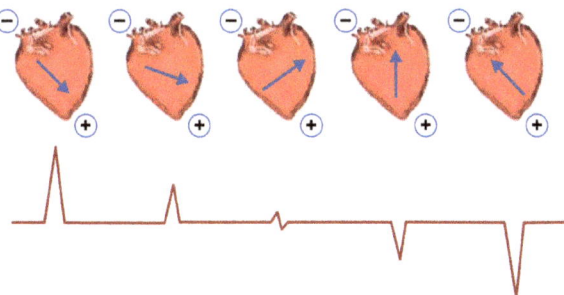

Fig. 8: Formation of waves—biphasic deflection.

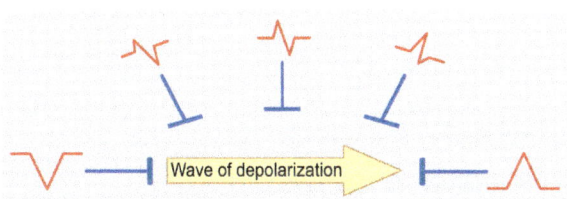

Fig. 9: Waves of depolarization.

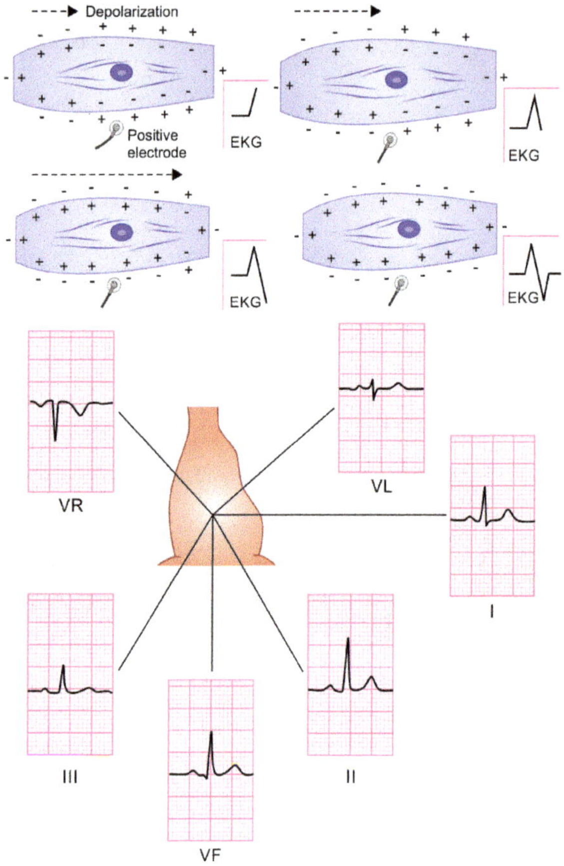

Chapter 2: Technical Aspects of ECG

Fig. 10: Formation of different waveforms.

Precordial Leads

Placement and electrocardiogram of precordial leads have been shown in **Figures 11 to 13**.

Color Codes Given by AHA

The color codes given by AHA have been shown in **Figure 14**.

Chapter 2: Technical Aspects of ECG

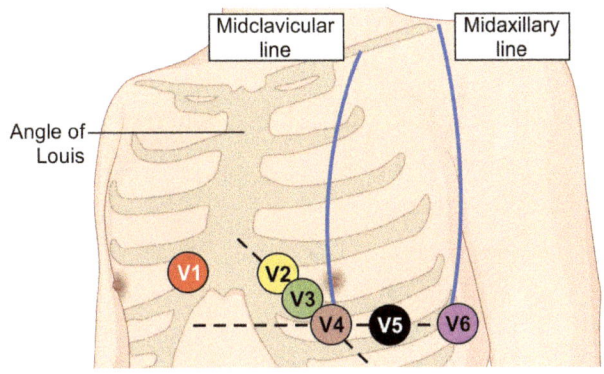

Fig. 11: Placement of precordial leads.

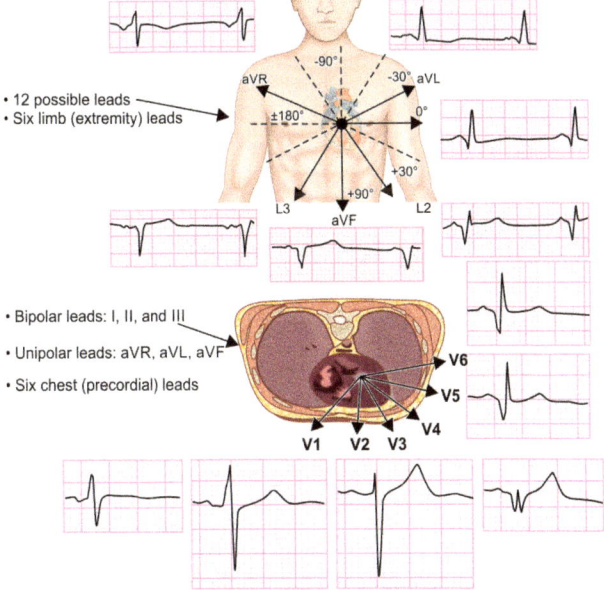

- 12 possible leads
- Six limb (extremity) leads

- Bipolar leads: I, II, and III
- Unipolar leads: aVR, aVL, aVF
- Six chest (precordial) leads

Fig. 12: Twelve-possible precordial leads along with ECG.

Chapter 2: Technical Aspects of ECG

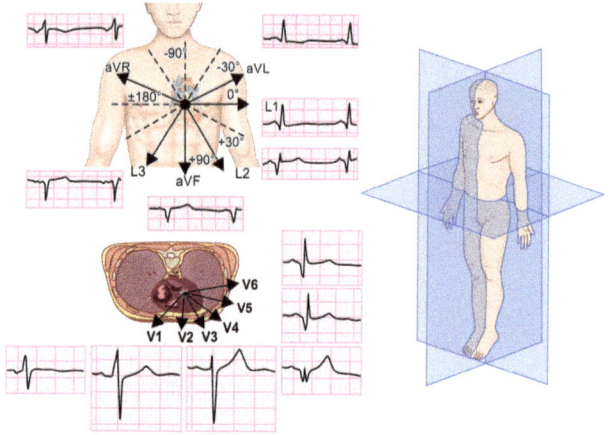

Fig. 13: Twelve-possible leads and their ECG.

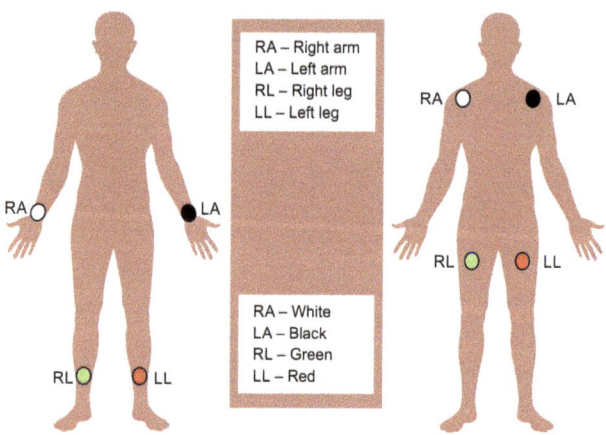

Fig. 14: Color codes given by AHA.

Limb Leads Electrodes

- Right arm
- Left arm
- Left leg **(Fig. 15)**

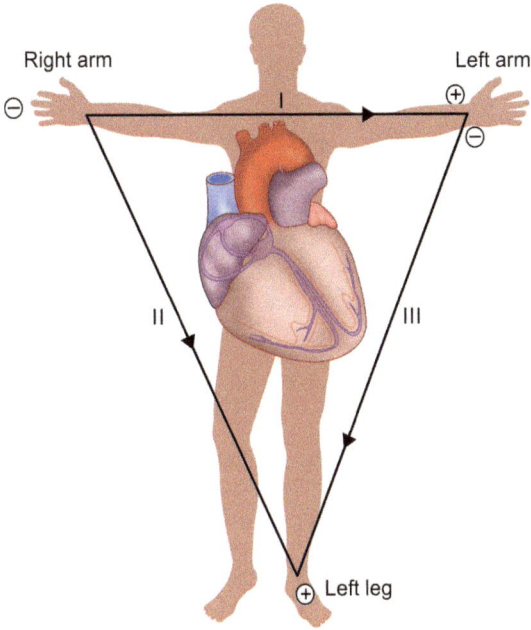

Fig. 15: Limb leads electrodes.

Lead I:
- Lead one "travels" horizontally
- Its left pole (LA) is positive and its right pole (RA) is negative. Therefore, lead I = LA minus RA.
- Lead I is conventionally constructed such that the left arm electrode is attached to the positive pole of the galvanometer and the right arm to the negative pole.
- Shows a positive wave when an impulse moves towards the left arm and a negative wave when an impulse moves away from the left arm **(Fig. 16)**.

Lead II:
- Lead II points downward diagonally
- The left leg is attached to the positive pole and the right arm to the negative pole

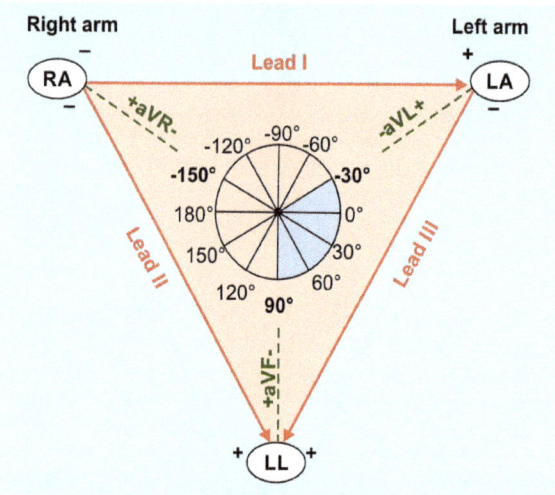

Fig. 16: Lead I, II and III.

- Lower pole (LL) is positive and upper pole (RA) is negative **(Fig. 16)**
- Lead II = LL minus RA

Lead III:
- Lead III points downward diagonally
- The left leg is attached to the positive pole and the left arm to the negative pole
- Lower pole (LL) is positive and upper pole (LA) is negative **(Fig. 16)**
- Lead III = LL minus LA

Bipolar leads:

Bipolar leads are shown in **Figure 17**.

Unipolar or Augmented Limb Leads

Record the electrical voltages at one location rather than relative to the voltage at another electrode.

- Lead aVR: The unipolar electrode is positioned over the right arm and is capable of detecting the flow of electrical impulse directed toward the right shoulder. The location of aVR is –150 degrees.

Chapter 2: Technical Aspects of ECG

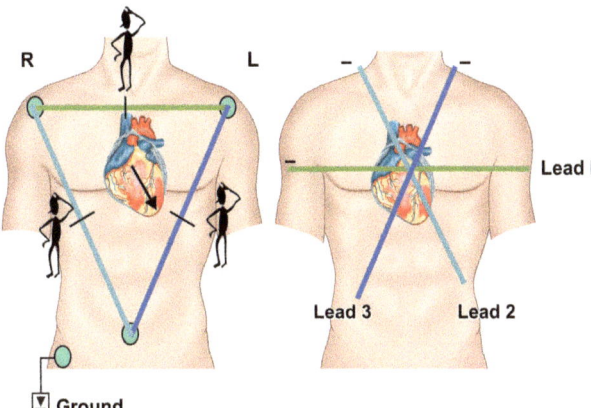

Fig. 17: Bipolar leads.

- Lead aVL: The unipolar electrode is positioned over the left arm and is capable of detecting potentials directed toward the left shoulder. The location of aVL is −30 degrees.
- Lead aVF: The unipolar electrode is positioned over the left leg and is capable of detecting potentials directed toward the left groin. The location of aVF is +90 degrees **(Fig. 18)**

All 12 Leads

All 12 leads are shown in **Figure 19**.

Arrangement of Leads

Anatomic groups:
Arrangement of leads in anatomic groups is shown in **Figure 20**.

Lead Placement

Standard Leads (Bipolar)
- I: Lateral wall
- II: Inferior wall
- III: Inferior wall

Augmented Leads (Unipolar)
- aVR: No mans land
- aVL: Lateral wall
- aVF: Inferior wall

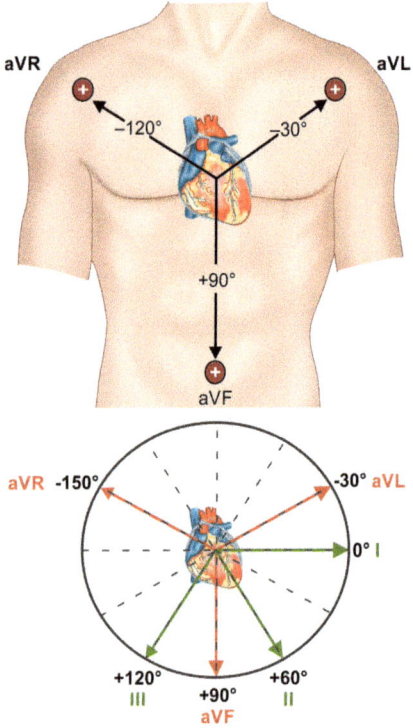

Fig. 18: Unipolar or augmented limb leads.

Chest Leads (Unipolar)
- V1: Septal wall
- V2: Septal wall
- V3: Anterior wall
- V4: Anterior wall
- V5: Lateral wall
- V6: Lateral wall

Chapter 2: Technical Aspects of ECG

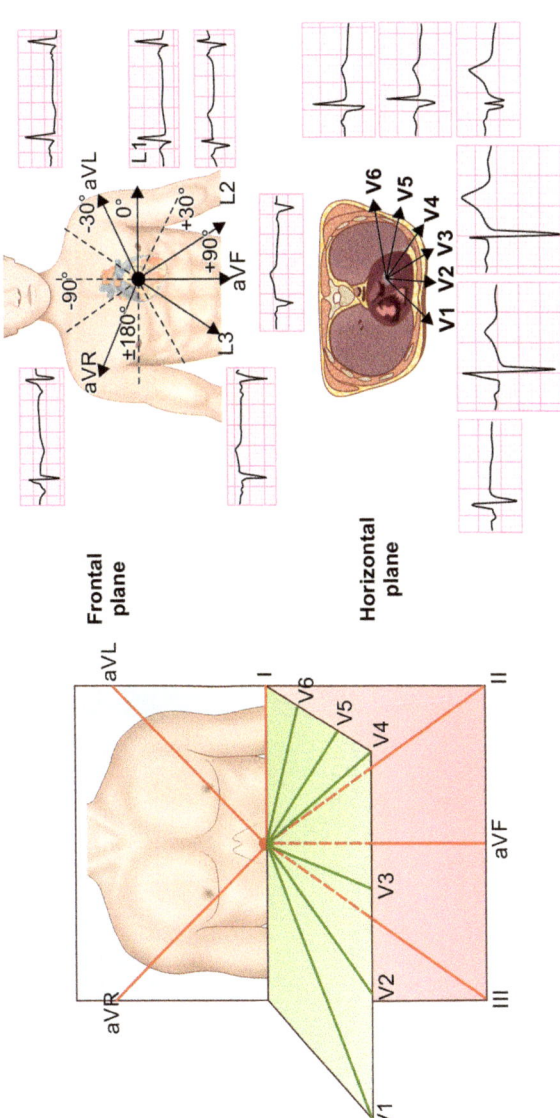

Fig. 19: All 12 leads.

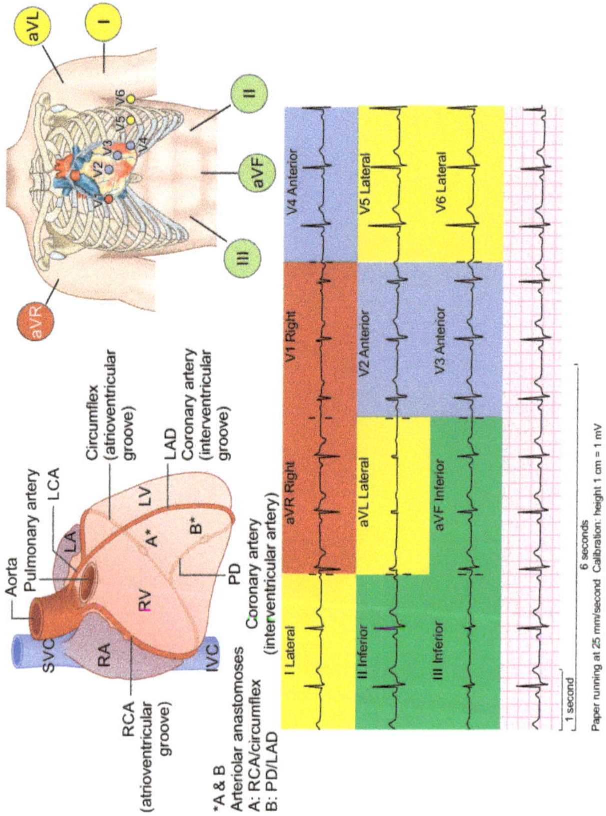

Chapter 2: Technical Aspects of ECG

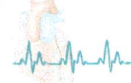

Fig. 20: Arrangement of leads.

Chapter 2: Technical Aspects of ECG

Ambulatory ECG Monitoring

Indications
- Unexplained recurrent syncope, near syncope, or episodic dizziness
- Unexplained recurrent palpitations **(Box 1)**

Holter Monitor/Loop Recorder
- Holter monitoring involves a continuous recording of the cardiac electrical activity for a period of 24–48 hours.
- The device consists of a small, battery-operated recorder that continuously records the cardiac electrical activity from the electrodes placed on the patient's chest **(Fig. 21)**.

Information on the ECG
- Patient's demographics
- Note the speed of the ECG strip
- Determine the heart rate
- Determine the rhythm
- Determine QRS axis
- Check the individual waves, calculate the intervals and look for any abnormalities

Determining the correct placement of the ECG leads:
- Limb leads
    - aVR is always negative
    - Lead I is always positive
    - Lead II, III is positive or biphasic

Box 1: Ambulatory ECG monitor type.

- Continuous ECG monitor (i.e., Holter monitor)
- Event (loop) monitor
- Patch monitor
- Mobile cardiac outpatient telemetry (MCOT)
- Implantable loop recorder
- Commercially available heart rate monitor (e.g., wristbands, smart watches)
- Commercially available heart rhythm monitors (e.g., smart watches, hand-held devices, smartphone-based electrode cards, etc.)

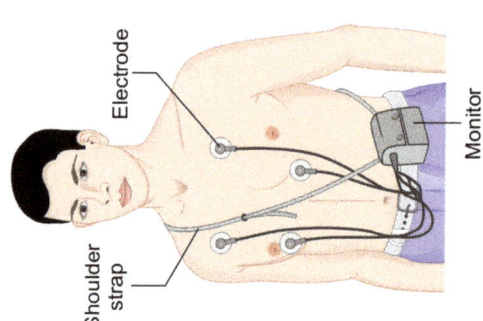
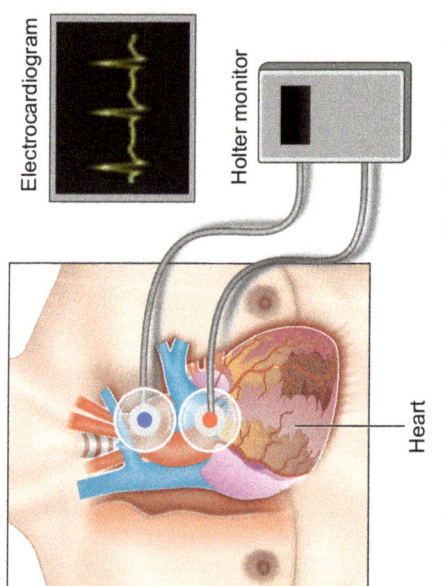

Fig. 21: Holter monitor.

Chapter 2: Technical Aspects of ECG

Precordial lead configurations

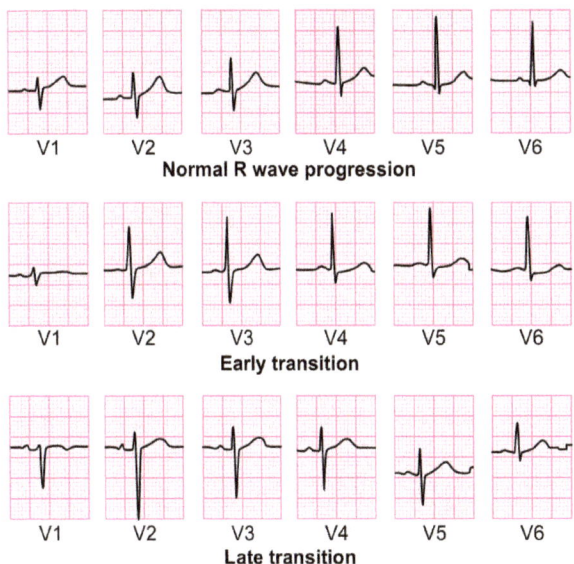

Fig. 22: Precordial lead configurations.

- Chest leads
  - Look at the R wave progression. The normal R wave progression and its abnormalities are summarized in **Figure 22.**

Lead Reversal ECG

Lead reversal ECG is shown in **Figure 23**.

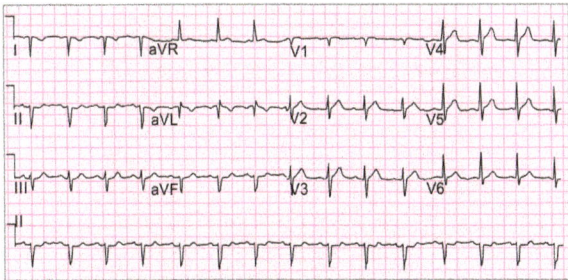

Fig. 23: Electrocardiogram showing lead reversal.

Chapter 2: Technical Aspects of ECG

PROCEDURE OF OBTAINING AN ECG: A STEP BY STEP CHECKLIST

- Gather the necessary equipment:
  - ECG machine
  - Self-adhesive ECG electrodes—to attach the ECG leads to the patient.
  - Razor—may be required to remove hair to provide adequate electrode contact with the skin.
- Confirm the patient's name and date of birth.
- Briefly explain the following to the patient: "I need to record an ECG which is an electrical trace of your heart. The procedure will involve placing some sticky pads onto your chest and limbs. I will then connect these sticky pads to the ECG machine's leads to record the tracing."
- If the patient is a female, explain the need for a chaperone: "One of the female ward staff members will be present throughout the procedure, acting as a chaperone, would that be alright?"
- Adequately expose the patient's chest for the procedure (offer a blanket to allow exposure only when required). Exposing the patient's lower limbs and wrists is also mandatory to apply the limb leads.
- Ask the patient to lay on the clinical examination couch with the head of the couch at a 45° angle.
- Count the intercostal spaces by palpation.

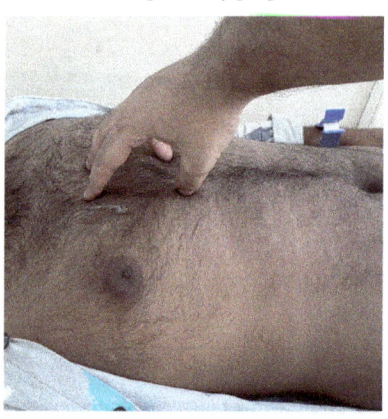

Electrode Placement

- A 12-lead ECG consists of 10 electrodes, 6 on the chest and 4 on the limbs.
- It is important to ensure each electrode has good skin contact, which may involve cleaning or shaving the areas where you need to place electrodes.

Chest electrode and lead placement (V1–V6)

Apply the six chest electrodes in the following locations:

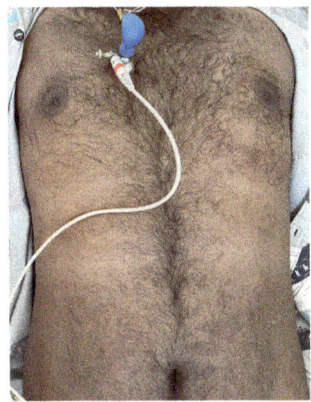

- V1: 4th intercostal space at the right sternal edge.

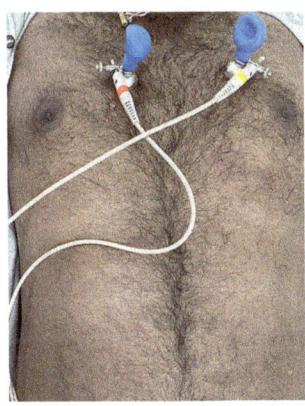

- V2: 4th intercostal space at the left sternal edge.

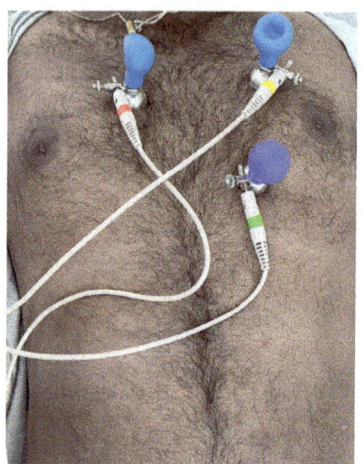

- V3: Midway between the V2 and V4 electrodes.

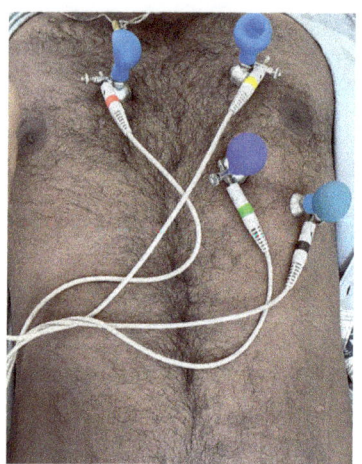

- V4: 5th intercostal space in the midclavicular line.

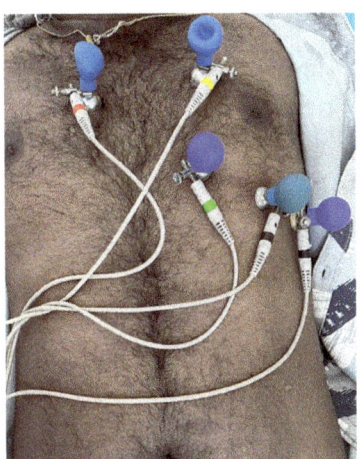

- V5: Left anterior axillary line at the same horizontal level as V4.

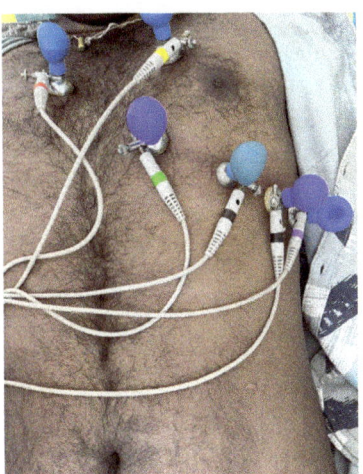

- V6: Left mid-axillary line at the same horizontal level as V4 and V5.

Chapter 2: Technical Aspects of ECG

Limb Electrode and Lead Placement

Apply the four limb electrodes on a distal bony prominence in the following locations:

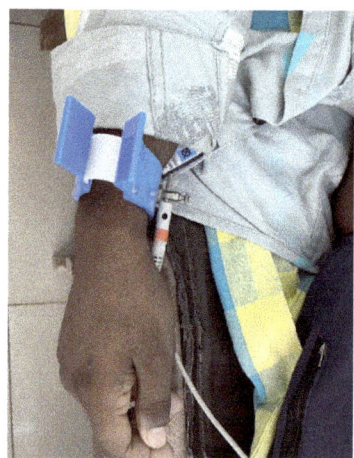

- Red (RA): On the ulnar styloid process of the right arm.

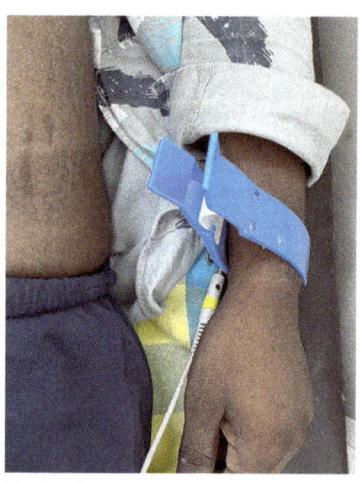

- Yellow (LA): On the ulnar styloid process of the left arm.

Chapter 2: Technical Aspects of ECG

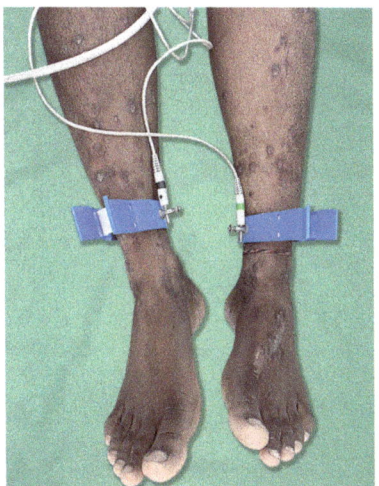

- Green (LL): On the medial or lateral malleolus of the left leg.
- Black (RL): On the medial or lateral malleolus of the right leg.

Use the mnemonic "Ride Your Green Bike" useful for remembering the placement of the limb leads, starting clockwise from the right wrist.

Recording the ECG Trace

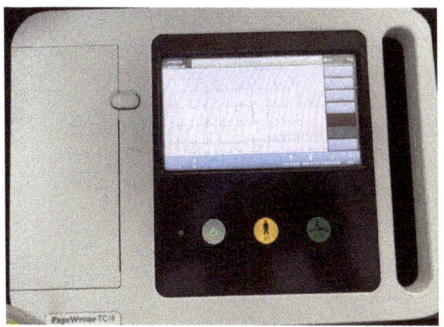

1. Turn the ECG machine on and ensure ECG paper has been loaded into the machine.

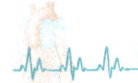
Chapter 2: Technical Aspects of ECG

2. Confirm all the electrodes are attached in the appropriate locations.
3. Kindly ask the patient to remain still and quiet during the recording as muscle activity can interfere with the ECG trace.
4. Press the appropriate button on the ECG machine to record the ECG trace.

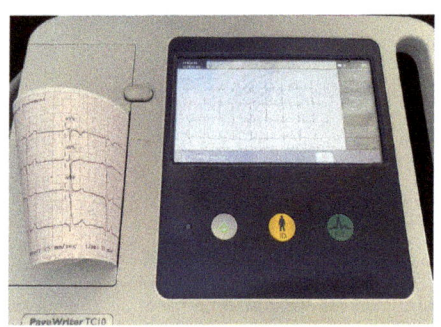

Completion of Procedure

- Once an ECG trace has been obtained, switch off the ECG machine.
- Gently remove the ECG Leads
- Explain to the patient that the procedure is now complete.
- Label the ECG with the patient's details:
  - Name, Age and Gender
  - Date of Birth
  - Hospital number
- Document your findings in the patient's notes.

Rate, Rhythm, and Axis

CHAPTER 3

READING 12-LEAD ECG

The best way to read 12-lead electrocardiogram (ECG) is to develop a step-by-step approach.

We present a 7-step approach:
1. Calculate the **rate**
2. Determine **rhythm**
3. Determine QRS **axis**
4. Examine individual **waves**
5. Calculate **intervals**
6. Assess for **hypertrophy**
7. Look for evidence of **infarction**/other **pathology**.

RATE

Rule of 300

Option 1:
- Count the number of "big boxes" between two QRS complexes and divide this into 300 (smaller boxes with 1,500) **(Fig. 1)**
- For regular rhythms.

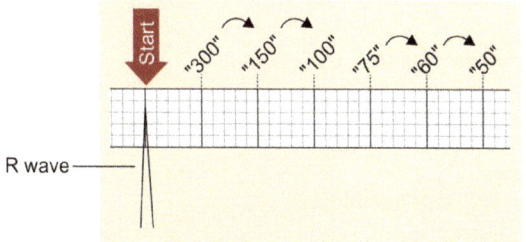

Fig. 1: Rule of 300.

Chapter 3: Rate, Rhythm, and Axis

Table 1: Calculation of rate with rule of 300.

No. of big boxes	Rate
1	300
2	150
3	100
4	75
5	60
6	50

Option 2:
- Find an R wave that lands on a bold line.
- Count the number of large boxes to the next R wave. If the second R wave is 1 large box away the rate is 300, 2 boxes-150, 3 boxes-100, 4 boxes-75, etc.

It may be easiest to memorize Table 1.

Calculating rate:

As a general interpretation, look at **lead II** at the bottom part of the ECG strip. This lead is the **rhythm strip,** which shows the rhythm for the whole time the ECG is recorded. Look at the number of squares between one RR intervals. To calculate the rate, use any of the following formulas:

$$\text{Rate} = \frac{300}{\text{Number of big squares between R-R interval}}$$

OR

$$\text{Rate} = \frac{1,500}{\text{Number of small squares between R-R interval}}$$

For example (**Fig. 2**):

$$\text{Rate} = \frac{300}{3} \text{ OR } \frac{1,500}{15}$$

Rate = 100 beats per minute

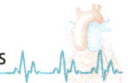

Chapter 3: Rate, Rhythm, and Axis

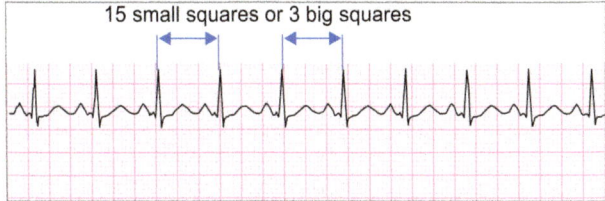

Fig. 2: Calculating heart rate by using small squares/big squares.

6-Second Rule

- ECGs record 6 seconds of rhythm per page
- Count the number of beats present on the ECG
- Multiply by 10

For Irregular Rhythms

If you think that the rhythm is not regular, count the number of electrical beats in a 6-second strip and multiply that number by 10 (note that some ECG strips have 3 seconds and 6 seconds marks).

Example below (Fig. 3):

There are 8 waves in this 6-second strip.

Rate = (Number of waves in 6-second strips) × 10
    =   8 × 10
    =   **80** bpm

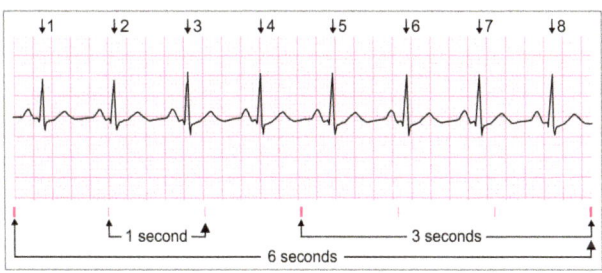

Fig. 3: Calculating heart rate by using 6-second strip.

Chapter 3: Rate, Rhythm, and Axis

Table 2: Causes for bradycardia and tachycardia.

Interpretation	Bpm	Causes
Normal	60–100	–
Bradycardia	<60	Hypothermia, increased vagal tone (due to vagal stimulation, e.g., drugs), athletes, hypothyroidism, beta-blockade, marked intracranial hypertension, obstructive jaundice, and even in uremia, structural SA node disease, or ischemia
Tachycardia	>100	Any cause of adrenergic stimulation (including pain); thyrotoxicosis; hypovolemia; vagolytic drugs (e.g., atropine) anemia, pregnancy; vasodilator drugs, including many hypotensive agents; fever, myocarditis

RHYTHM

Determine Regularity

- Look at the R-R distances (using a caliper or markings on a pen or paper) **(Fig. 4)**.
- Regular (are they equidistant apart)? Occasionally irregular? Regularly irregular? Irregularly irregular?
- Look at p waves and their relationship to QRS complexes.
- Lead II is commonly used
- Regular or irregular?
- If in doubt, use a **calipers or paper strip** to map out consecutive beats and see whether the rate is the same further along with the ECG **(Figs. 5A and B)**.
- Measure ventricular rhythm by measuring the R-R interval and atrial rhythm by measuring the P-P interval **(Figs. 5A and B)**.

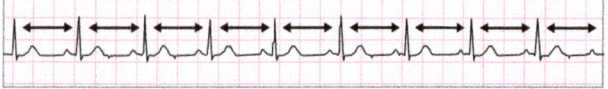

Fig. 4: Electrocardiogram strip showing regularity.

Chapter 3: Rate, Rhythm, and Axis

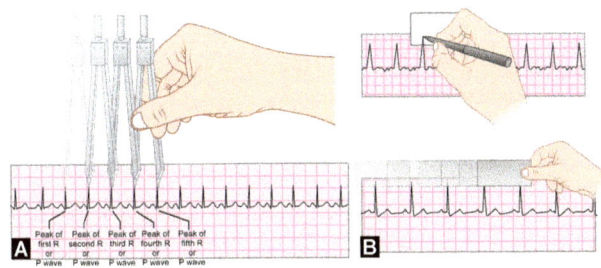

Figs. 5A and B: (A) Caliper method; (B) Paper and pen method.

Normal Sinus Rhythm—P Wave followed by QRS

Normal sinus rhythm is shown in **Figure 6**.

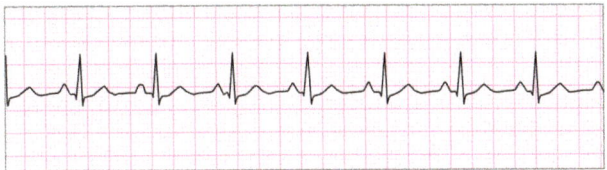

Fig. 6: Electrocardiogram showing normal sinus rhythm.

Sinus Bradycardia

Sinus bradycardia is shown in **Figure 7.**
   Rate <60 bpm, otherwise normal

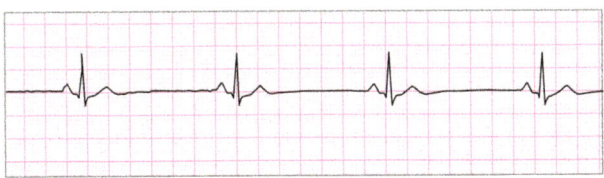

Fig. 7: Electrocardiogram showing sinus bradycardia.

Sinus Tachycardia

Sinus tachycardia is shown in **Figure 8**.
Rate >100 bpm, otherwise, normal

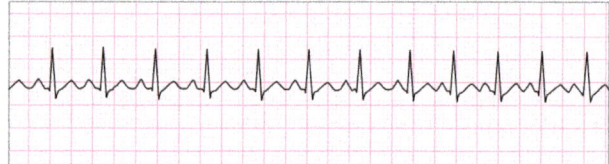

Fig. 8: Electrocardiogram showing sinus tachycardia.

Sinus Pause

Sinus pause is shown in **Figure 9**.

In disease (e.g., sick sinus syndrome), the SA node can fail in its pacing function. If failure is brief and recovery is prompt, the result is only a missed beat (sinus pause). If recovery is delayed and no other focus assumes pacing function, cardiac arrest follows.

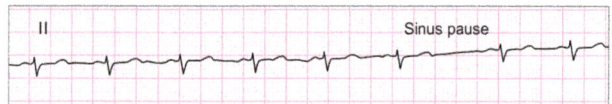

Fig. 9: Electrocardiogram showing sinus pause.

Atrial Fibrillation

Atrial fibrillation is shown in **Figure 10**.

Atrial fibrillation is the most common cardiac arrhythmia involving atria. Rate = ~150 bpm, irregularly irregular, baseline irregularity, no visible p waves, QRS occur irregularly with its length usually <0.12 seconds.

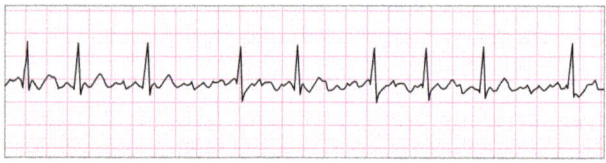

Fig. 10: Electrocardiogram showing atrial fibrillation.

Chapter 3: Rate, Rhythm, and Axis

Atrial Flutter

Atrial flutter is shown in **Figure 11**.

❖ Atrial rate = ~300 bpm, similar to atrial fibrillation, but have flutter waves, ECG baseline adapts "saw-toothed" appearance.
❖ Occurs with atrioventricular block (fixed degree), e.g., 3 flutters to 1 QRS complex.

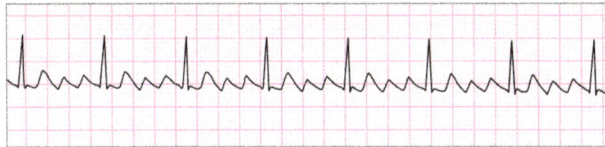

Fig. 11: Electrocardiogram showing atrial flutter.

Ventricular Fibrillation

Ventricular fibrillation is shown in **Figure 12**.

A severely abnormal heart rhythm (arrhythmia) can be life-threatening. Emergency—requires basic life support. Rate cannot be discerned, rhythm is unorganized.

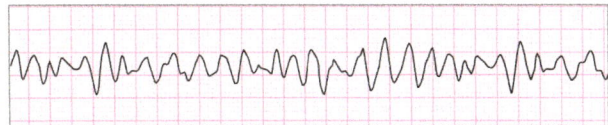

Fig. 12: Electrocardiogram showing ventricular fibrillation.

Ventricular Tachycardia

Ventricular tachycardia is shown in **Figure 13**.

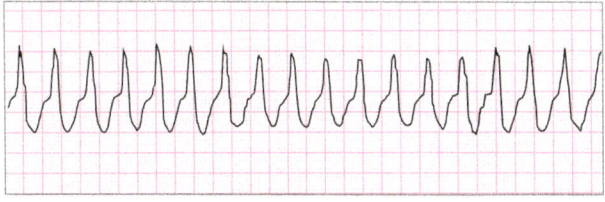

Fig. 13: Electrocardiogram showing ventricular tachycardia.

Fast heart rhythm that originates in one of the ventricles—potentially life-threatening arrhythmia because it may lead to ventricular fibrillation, asystole, and sudden death. Rate = 100–250 bpm.

Torsades de Pointes

Torsades de pointes is shown in **Figure 14**.

Literally meaning twisting of points is a distinctive form of polymorphic ventricular tachycardia characterized by a gradual change in the amplitude and twisting of the QRS complexes around the isoelectric line. Rate cannot be determined.

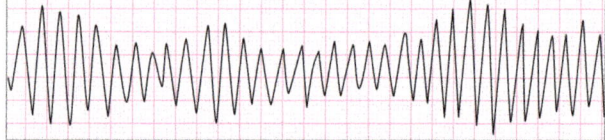

Fig. 14: Electrocardiogram showing Torsades de pointes.

Supraventricular Tachycardia

Supraventricular tachycardia (SVT) is shown in **Figure 15.**

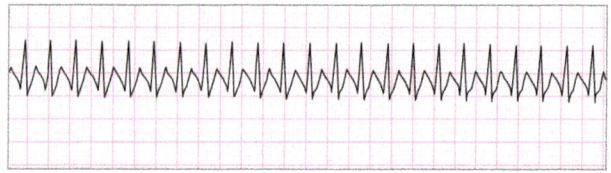

Fig. 15: Electrocardiogram showing supraventricular tachycardia.

Supraventricular tachycardia is any tachycardic rhythm originating above the ventricular tissue. Atrial and ventricular rate = 150–250 bpm regular rhythm, p is usually not discernible.

AXIS

The QRS Axis

❖ The QRS axis represents overall direction of the heart's electrical activity.

Chapter 3: Rate, Rhythm, and Axis

- Abnormalities hint at:
    - Ventricular enlargement
    - Conduction blocks (i.e., hemiblocks)

Cardiac Axis

The cardiac axis refers to the general direction of the heart's depolarization wavefront (or mean electrical vector) in the frontal plane. With a healthy conducting system, the cardiac axis is related to where the major muscle bulk of the heart lies **(Fig. 16)**.

Electrical impulse that travels toward the electrode produces an upright (positive) deflection (of the QRS complex) relative to the isoelectric baseline. One that travels away produces negative deflection. And one that travels at a right angle to the lead produces a biphasic wave.

Determining the Axis

- The quadrant approach
- The equiphasic approach
- The classical method

The Quadrant Approach

Examine the QRS complex in leads I and aVF to determine if they are predominantly positive or predominantly negative. The combination should place the axis into one of the four quadrants below.

1. If net QRS in both I and aVF are positive → then its normal axis
2. If QRS in I is negative ad aVF is positive—that means they are **R**EACHING to each other → Axis is **R**IGHT

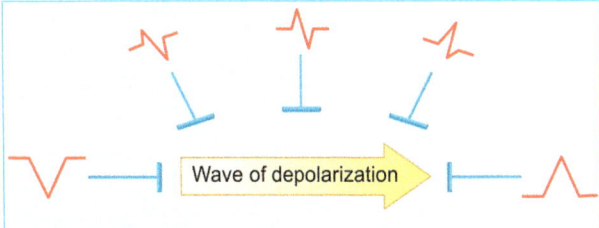

Fig. 16: Wave of depolarization shape of QRS complex in any lead depends on orientation of that lead to vector of depolarization.

3. If QRS in I is positive and aVF is negative: that means they are LEAVING to each other → Axis is **LEFT**
4. If net QRS in both I and aVF is negative → then its extreme axis/axis in No man's land **(Fig. 17)**.

Cardiac axis:

Different cardiac axes are shown in **Figures 18 to 20**.

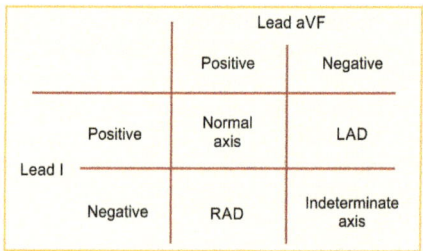

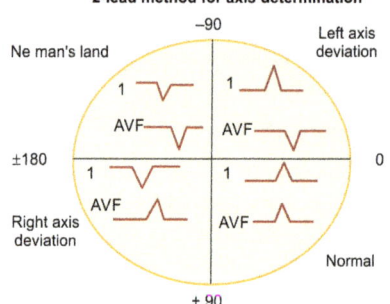

Fig. 17: The quadrant approach.

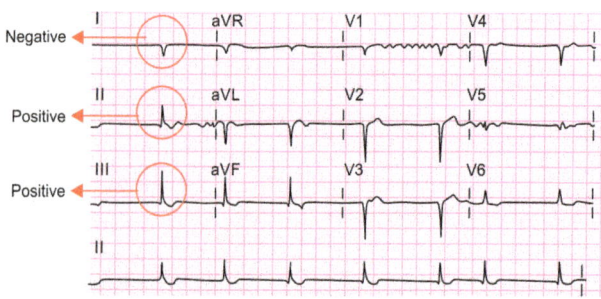

Fig. 18: Right axis deviation.

Chapter 3: Rate, Rhythm, and Axis

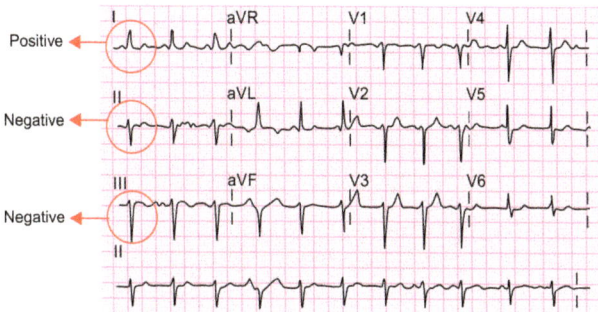

Fig. 19: Left axis deviation.

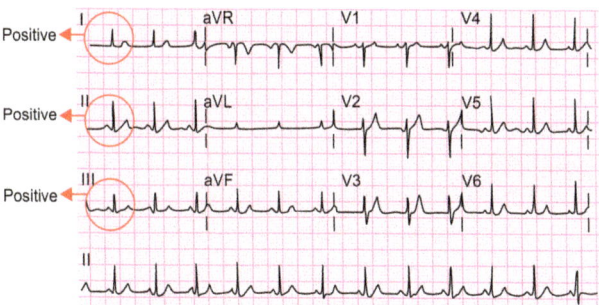

Fig. 20: Normal axis deviation.

Using leads I, II, III:

Using leads I, II and III has been explained in **Table 3**.

Table 3: Using leads I, II, and III.			
	Lead I	*Lead II*	*Lead III*
Normal	Upright	Upright	Upright
Physiological left axis	Upright	Upright/biphasic	Negative
Pathological left axis	Upright	Negative	Negative
Right axis	Negative	Upright/biphasic/negative	Upright
Extreme right axis	Negative	Negative	Negative

Causes of left axis deviation:

❖ Causes of left axis deviation are shown in **Box 1**.

> **Box 1:** Causes of left axis deviation.
>
> **Common causes of LAD (−30 to −90 degree):**
> - Left anterior hemiblock
> - LBBB
> - Left ventricular hypertrophy
> - Q waves of inferior myocardial infarction
> - Artificial cardiac pacing
> - Emphysema
> - Hyperkalemia
> - Wolff-Parkinson-White syndrome—right-sided accessory pathway
> - Tricuspid atresia
> - Ostium primum ASD
> - May be normal in the elderly and very obese
> - Due to high diaphragm during pregnancy, ascites, or abdominal tumors

Causes of right axis deviation:

Causes of right axis deviation are shown in **Box 2**.

> **Box 2:** Common causes of RAD (+110 to +180 degree).
>
> - Normal finding in children and tall thin adults
> - Right ventricular hypertrophy
> - Chronic lung disease even without pulmonary hypertension
> - Anterolateral myocardial infarction
> - Left posterior hemiblock
> - Pulmonary embolus
> - Wolff-Parkinson-White syndrome—left-sided accessory pathway
> - Atrial septal defect (ostium secundum)
> - Ventricular septal defect

Chapter 3: Rate, Rhythm, and Axis

Axis—extreme axis/Northwest territory:

Box 3 shows the extreme axis/Northwest territory.

> **Box 3:** Axis—extreme axis/Northwest territory
> (−180 to −90 degree).
>
> - Both I and aVF −ve = axis in the NORTHWEST TERRITORY
> - Causes of "No man's land"
>   - Dextrocardia
>   - Emphysema
>   - Hyperkalemia
>   - Lead transposition
>   - Artificial cardiac pacing
>   - Ventricular tachycardia

Undetermined axis:

When all extremity leads are biphasic, the axis is directed to the front or back, in a transverse plane. The axis is then undetermined.

CARDIAC AXIS THUMB RULE

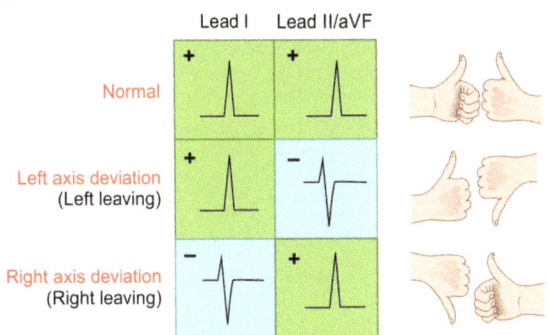

Cardiac axis thumb rule

Both thumbs are *up*
- ECG—if QRS in lead I and II are both positive
- Interpretation—normal

Thumbs *left* each other
- ECG—if QRS in lead I is up (+ve) and in lead II is down (-ve)
- Interpretation—left axis deviation

Thumbs are *right* towards each other
- ECG—if QRS in lead I is down (-ve) and in lead II is up (+ve)
- Interpretation—right axis deviation

Both thumbs are *down*
- ECG—if both lead I and II are negative
- Interpretation—right superior axis deviation (extreme right axis deviation).

Waves, Segments, and Intervals

CHAPTER 4

UNDERSTANDING ECG WAVEFORM

The best way to interpret an ECG is to do it step-by-step.

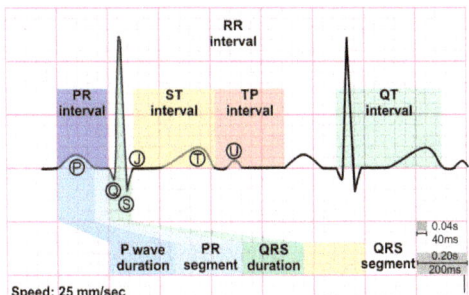

Fig. 1: Waves, segments and intervals in ECG.

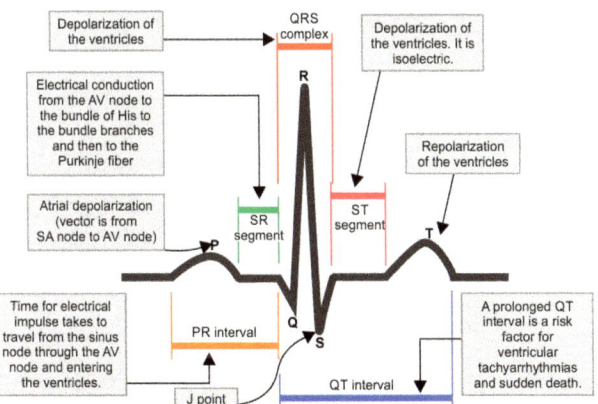

Fig. 2: Genesis of waves in ECG.

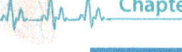

Chapter 4: Waves, Segments, and Intervals

P WAVES

Assess the P waves

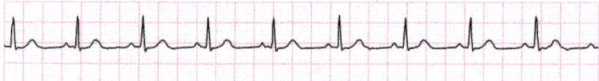

Fig. 3: P waves.

- Always positive in leads I, II, aVF, and V3, V6 with P axis in frontal plane is between 0° and +75° **(Fig. 3)**
- Commonly biphasic in lead V1
- Always negative in lead aVR
- The initial portion is due to RA depolarization and the late portion is due to LA depolarization. The duration of RA depolarization is 0.02–0.04 seconds and that of LA is 0.05–0.06 seconds.
- <2.5 small squares in duration and <2.5 small squares in amplitude
- Best seen in leads II

Abnormalities of P Wave

Abnormalities of P wave are shown in **Figure 4**.

Right Atrial Enlargement

- Tall (>2.5 mm), pointed P waves (P pulmonale) **(Fig. 5)**
- Seen in chronic obstructive pulmonary disease (COPD), cor pulmonale, and atrial septal defects (ASD)

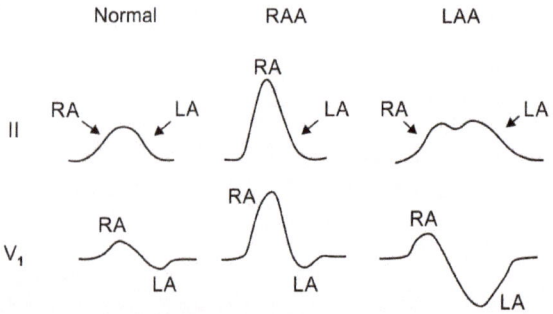

Fig. 4: Abnormalities of P wave.

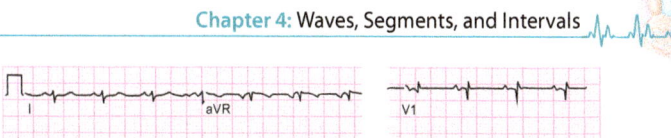

Fig. 5: Right atrial enlargement.

Left Atrial Enlargement (Fig. 6)

- Notched/bifid ("M" shaped) P wave (P "mitrale") in limb leads
- Double-peaked-like bent staple or camel-humped appearance
- Seen with mitral stenosis, mitral regurgitation, and systemic hypertension

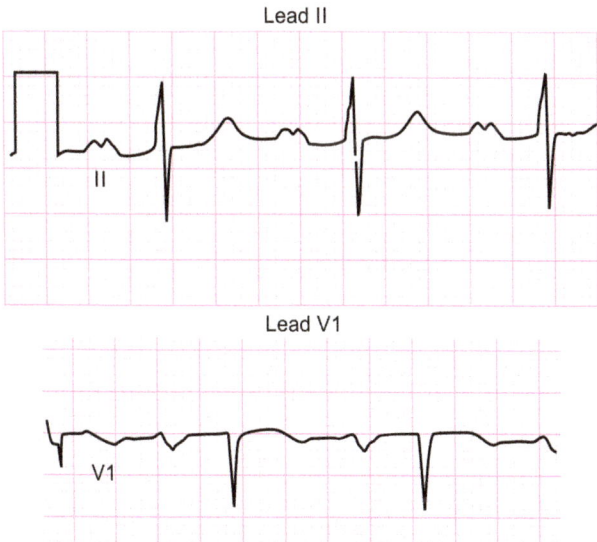

Fig. 6: Left atrial enlargement.

Other P Wave Abnormalities

- In Ebstein's anomaly you can see very tall P waves called as Himalayan **P** waves.
- **Inverted P wave** is seen in dextrocardia.
- In sick sinus syndrome, the P wave morphology keeps on changing or sometimes it can be absent also.
- **Absent P waves** in regular rhythm: In SA block and AV junctional rhythm.
- In atrial fibrillation P waves are absent and they are replaced by fibrillary **waves.** If the size of the fibrillatory f waves is >1 mm (coarse atrial fibrillation), is suggestive of LAE.
- In atrial flutter, there is regular rhythm but P waves are replaced by saw-tooth appearing waves called **flutter waves**.
- **Polymorphic P waves:** Three or more different P wave morphologies in the same lead, consider multifocal atrial tachycardia.
- **Biatrial enlargement:** Diphasic P in V1 or tall-peaked P in V1 with notched P in V5 or V6.

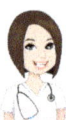

Nursing Considerations

Observe patient for atrial arrhythmias like atrial flutter and fibrillation. Patients with atrial fibrillation are prescribed with anticoagulant therapy to prevent stroke. Nurses have a prime responsibility to teach their patients about the importance of anticoagulant therapy, and the significance of PT/INR.

PR INTERVAL

- **(P wave + PR segment)**
- The PR interval is the time from the onset of the P wave to the start of the QRS complex.
- It includes:
    - Atrial depolarization
    - AV node conduction delay (0.07 s)
    - And the passage of impulse through the bundle of His and bundle branches

Chapter 4: Waves, Segments, and Intervals

- The normal PR interval is between 120 and 200 ms duration (3-5 small squares).

Atrioventricular Block

First Degree Heart (AV) Block

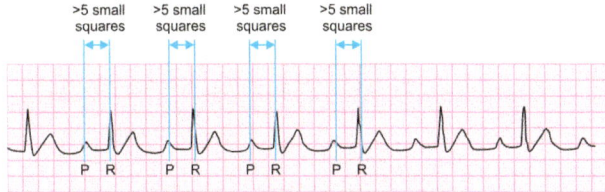

Fig. 7: First degree heart block.

- P wave precedes QRS complex but PR intervals prolong >0.20 s (>5 small squares) and remain constant from beat to beat **(Fig. 7)**.
- Normal QRS complexes both in duration and configuration
- Can be due to delay in AV node or His Purkinje system or both

Second Degree Heart Block

1. *Mobitz Type I or Wenckebach*

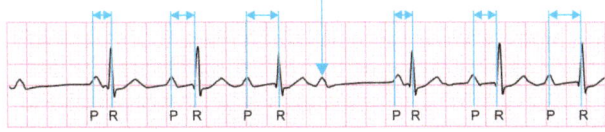

Fig. 8: Second degree heart block—Mobitz type I.

- Runs in cycle, first PR interval is often normal. With successive beat, PR interval lengthens until there will be a P wave with no following QRS complex.
- There is a progressive shortening of the RR interval until a P wave is blocked.
- The block is at AV node proximal to His bundle, often transient, may be asymptomatic **(Fig. 8)**.

Chapter 4: Waves, Segments, and Intervals

2. *Mobitz Type II*
   - PR interval is constant, duration is normal/prolonged.
   - Periodically, no conduction between atria and ventricles—producing a P wave with no associated QRS complex (blocked P wave).
   - The block is most often below AV node, at bundle of His or bundle block.
   - May progress to third degree heart block.
   - Mostly occurs in the setting of an acute anterior MI **(Fig. 9)**.

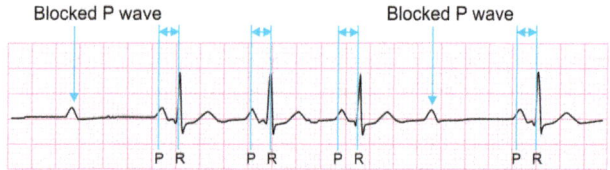

Fig. 9: Second degree heart block—Mobitz type II.

Third Degree Heart Block (Complete Heart Block)

- No relationship between P waves and QRS complexes **(Fig. 10)**.
- An accessory pacemaker in the lower chambers will typically activate the ventricles—escape rhythm.
- Atrial rate = 60–100 bpm. Ventricular rate based on site of the escape pacemaker. Atrial and ventricular rhythms both are regular.
- Complete AV block can be at the level of AV node (usually in the congenital causes), within the bundle of His or distal to it in the Purkinje system (in the acquired causes) **(Box 1)**.

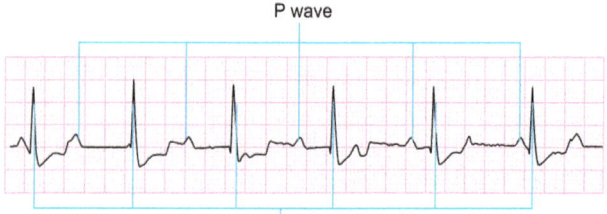

Fig. 10: Third degree heart block.

Chapter 4: Waves, Segments, and Intervals

> **Box 1:** Causes of heart block.

Congenital
Acquired
- Ischemia
- Degenerative process (Lenegre's disease, Lev's disease)
- Drugs (digitalis, quinidine, procainamide, beta blockers, calcium channel blockers)
- Rheumatic fever
- Myocarditis
- Hyperkalemia
- Cardiomyopathy (DCM)
- Chagas disease
- Diphtheria
- Infiltrative diseases—amyloidosis, sarcoidosis, scleroderma

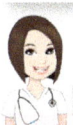

Nursing Considerations

- Lower-degree AV blocks are less likely to cause hemodynamic alterations and usually require only monitoring for progression. But as the AV block progresses, hemodynamic instability may lead to signs and symptoms and may need pacemaker insertion.
- Monitor closely the heart rate, symptoms of low cardiac output like syncope, decresed urine output, fatigue, loss of consciousness. The patient's medication use should be monitored closely.

Short PR Interval

A short PR interval is seen with: Pre-excitation syndromes (like Wolff–Parkinson–White syndrome or Lown–Ganong–Levine syndrome) and AV nodal (junctional) rhythm.

PR SEGMENT

- Isoelectric segment between the end of the P wave and the start of the QRS complex.
- PR segment depression is seen in pericarditis, atrial ischemia
- PR segment elevation can be seen in atrial ischemia
- PR elevation in lead aVR with ST depression is pathognomonic of acute pericarditis **(Fig. 11)**

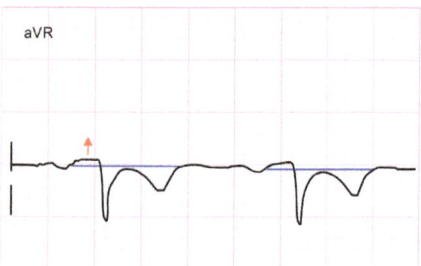

Fig. 11: PR segment.

QRS COMPLEX

QRS complex is the waveform immediately following the PR interval.

It consists of:

- Q wave: First negative deflection from the baseline following the P wave
- R wave: First positive deflection following the Q wave
- S wave: First negative deflection that extends below the baseline following the R wave

Q(q) Wave

- It is due to the initial depolarization of mid-portion of left side of the interventricular septum from left to right. Hence it is negative.
- Small "septal" Q waves are typically seen in the left-sided leads (I, aVL, V5, and V6) **(Fig. 12)**
- **Pathological Q wave:** Q wave prolongation (>0.04 s), > 2 mm deep and depression >25% of R wave is a manifestation of transmural myocardial necrosis **(Figs. 13 and 14)**.

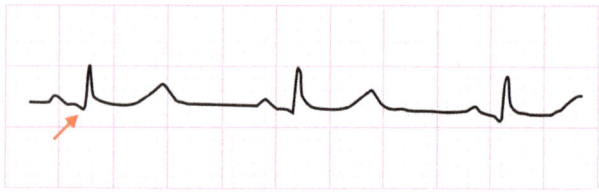

Fig. 12: Q waves.

Chapter 4: Waves, Segments, and Intervals

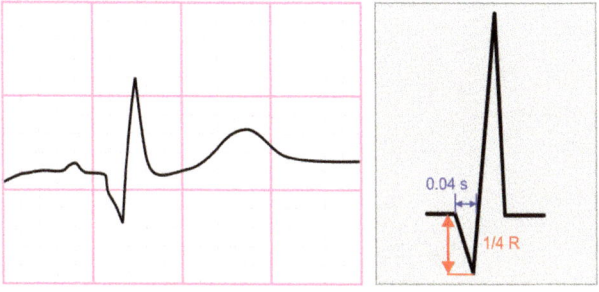

Fig. 13: Q wave prolongation.

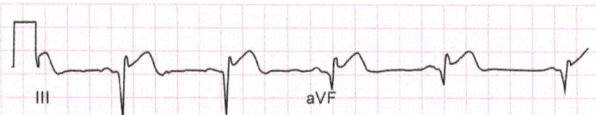

Fig. 14: ECG showing pathological Q wave.

- Other conditions with prominent Q waves are hypertrophic cardiomyopathy, infiltrative myocardial disease, and lead misplacement (upper limb leads placed on lower limbs)
- Absence of small septal Q waves in leads V5-6 is seen in LBBB.

R(r) Wave

- First positive deflection during ventricular depolarization
- The upper limit of R wave amplitude is 1.5 mV in lead I, 1.0 mV in lead aVL, 1.9 mV in leads II, III, and aVF, and 0.6 mV in V1.
- Among the precordial leads, the tallest R wave is seen in V4.
- R wave axis and criteria for chamber enlargement discussed separately.

S(s) Wave

- Negative deflection of ventricular depolarization that follows the first positive deflection (R)
- Due to the activation of last portion of the ventricular mass (posterior basal portion of LV, pulmonary conus, and uppermost portion of the interventricular septum)
- Duration of 0.01–0.02 seconds

Chapter 4: Waves, Segments, and Intervals

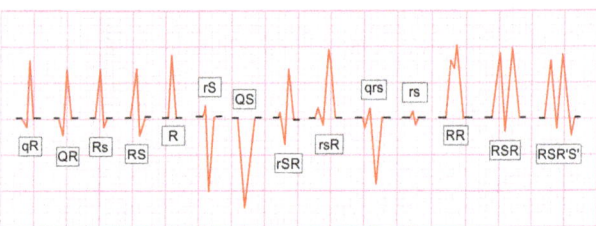

Fig. 15: Variation in QRS complex.

Variations in QRS Complexes

While the QRS is said to consist of positive deflections called R waves and negative deflections called Q and S waves, all three waves are not always seen **(Fig. 15)**.

- If there is no R wave, the complex is called a QS complex.
- If there is no Q wave, the complex is called a RS complex.

R'(r') Wave

Second positive deflection that may occur during ventricular depolarization following S wave.

Measuring the QRS Complex

- Starting point is where first wave of complex starts to move away from baseline.
- Ending point is where last wave of complex begins to level out (flatten) at, above, or below the baseline. Referred to as the J point **(Fig. 16)**.

LOW VOLTAGE QRS

- The amplitudes of all the QRS complexes in the limb leads are <5 mm; or the amplitudes of all the QRS complexes in the precordial leads are <10 mm **(Fig. 17)**.
- Causes are:
  - Obese patient
  - Restrictive cardiomyopathy
  - Pericardial effusion
  - Hypothyroid
  - Hypothermia
  - Myocarditis
  - Amyloidosis

Chapter 4: Waves, Segments, and Intervals

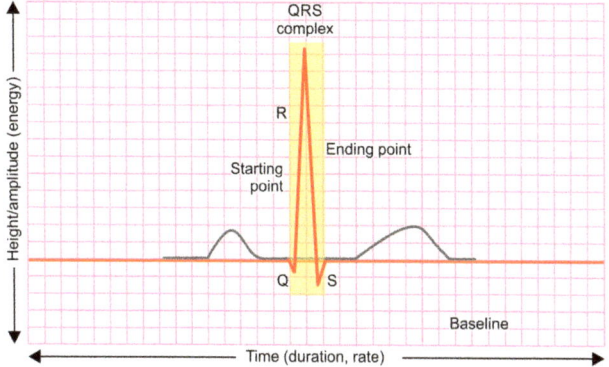

Fig. 16: Measuring QRS complex.

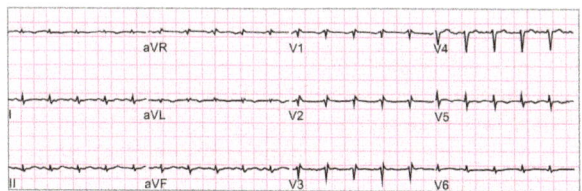

Fig. 17: Low voltage QRS.

HIGH VOLTAGE QRS COMPLEXES

This is seen with ventricular hypertrophy/chamber enlargement.

Right ventricular hypertrophy

Normally the R wave in lead V1 is less than S wave in the same lead. If R wave height is found to be more than S wave depth in lead V1 it is the voltage criteria for RVH **(Fig. 18)**.

- RAD (>110 degrees)
- Tall R-waves in V1
- R/S >1 in V1

Supporting criteria **(Fig. 19)**

- P pulmonale.
- Right ventricular strain pattern = ST depression/T wave inversion in the right precordial (V1-4) and inferior (II, III, aVF) leads.

Chapter 4: Waves, Segments, and Intervals

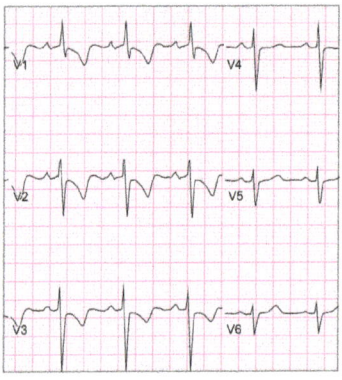

Fig. 18: Right ventricular hypertrophy—R/S in V1 >1.

- S1 S2 S3 pattern
- Deep S waves in the lateral leads (I, aVL, V5-V6) **(Fig. 19)**.

Left ventricular hypertrophy

To determine LVH, use one of the following criteria **(Fig. 20)**:

- **Sokolow and Lyon criteria**: S (V1) + R (V5 or V6) >35 mm
- **Cornell criteria**: S (V3) + R (aVL) >28 mm (men) or >20 mm (women)

Others: R (aVL) >13 mm

Causes of LVH and RVH are listed in **Table 1**.

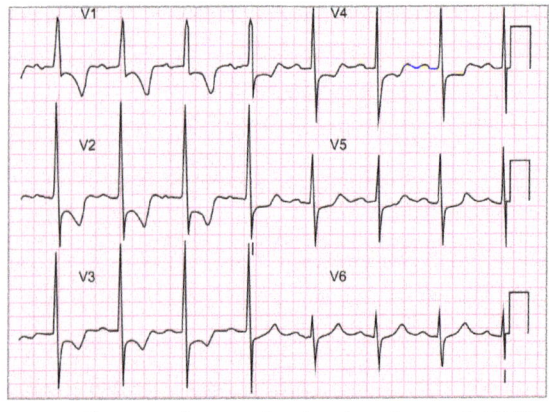

Fig. 19: Electrocardiogram showing deep S waves in V5, V6.

Chapter 4: Waves, Segments, and Intervals

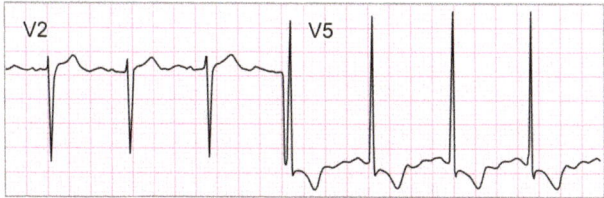

Fig. 20: Sokolow and Lyon criteria.

Table 1: Common causes of LVH and RVH.	
Causes of LVH	*Causes of RVH*
<ul><li>Hypertension (most common cause)</li><li>Aortic stenosis</li><li>Aortic regurgitation</li><li>Mitral regurgitation</li><li>Coarctation of the aorta</li><li>Hypertrophic cardiomyopathy</li></ul>	<ul><li>Pulmonary hypertension</li><li>Tetralogy of Fallot</li><li>Pulmonary valve stenosis</li><li>Ventricular septal defect (VSD)</li><li>Mitral stenosis</li><li>Pulmonary embolism (chronic)</li><li>COPD</li><li>Athletic heart syndrome</li></ul>

Bundle Branch Blocks

Depolarization of the bundle branches and Purkinje fibers are seen as the QRS complex on the ECG.

Therefore, a conduction block of the bundle branches would be reflected as a change in the QRS complex.

- QRS complex widens (>0.12 sec).
- QRS morphology changes (varies depending on ECG lead, and if it is a right vs. left bundle) **(branch block).**

Right Bundle Branch Blocks

They are like "Rabbit ears" **(Fig. 21)**
- Wide QRS complex
- Diagnostic shape (upright "rabbit ears") in those leads overlying the right ventricle, V1 and V2.

Left Bundle Branch Blocks

- Wide QRS complex
- Downward deflection in V1 and V2 (right ventricular leads)

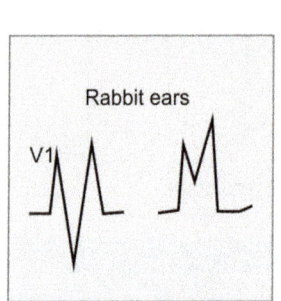
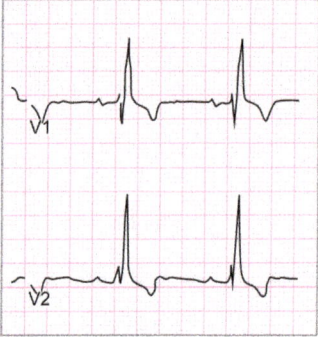

Fig. 21: Right bundle branch blocks.

❖ The QRS is upright and wide in V5 and V6 (may or may not be notched) **(Fig. 22)**.

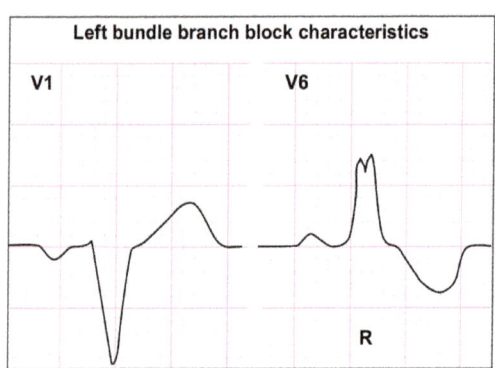

Fig. 22: Left bundle branch blocks.

Difference between LBBB and RBBB is shown in **Table 2**.

Table 2: Difference between LBBB and RBBB.	
Left bundle branch block (LBBB)	**Right bundle branch block (RBBB)**
Indirect activation causes left ventricle contracts later than the right ventricle.	Indirect activation causes right ventricle contracts later than the left ventricle.

Contd...

Contd...

Left bundle branch block (LBBB)	Right bundle branch block (RBBB)
QS or rS complex in V1—W-shaped RsR' wave in V6—M-shaped	Terminal R wave (rSR') in V1—M-shaped Slurred S wave in V6—W-shaped
Mnemonic: WILLIAM	Mnemonic: MARROW

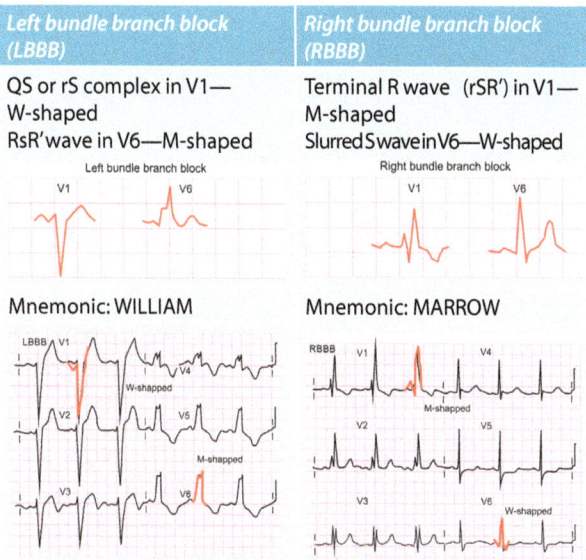

Right Bundle Branch Block

- Wide QRS, more than 120 ms (3 small squares)
- Broad notched R waves—rsr, rsR, or rSR' in V1, V2, V3, R, and wide R' >0.04s
- VAT in V1 >50 ms, but normal in V5, V6
- Other features include slurred S wave in lateral leads
- Minimum secondary ST-T changes in V1, V2 **(Fig. 23)**

Left Bundle Branch Block

- Wide QRS, more than 120 ms
- Broad notched R waves or rsR' in V5, V6, I, and aVL
- q waves absent in left-sided leads except aVL
- VAT in V5, V6 >0.06s, but normal in V1, V2
- Secondary ST-T changes in V5, V6, I, aVL

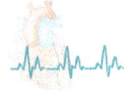

Chapter 4: Waves, Segments, and Intervals

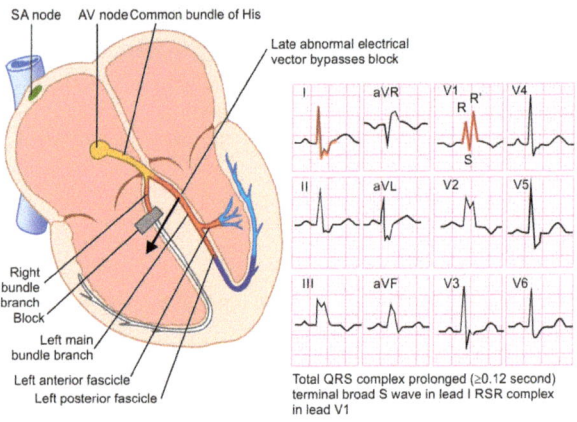

Fig. 23: QRS complex with right bundle branch block.

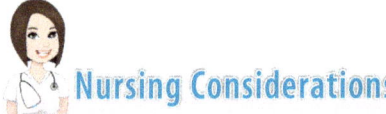

Nursing Considerations

Inform patients on the underlying causes of their illness and the importance of adherence to medical treatment.

J POINT

- Elevation or depression of the J point is seen with the various causes of ST segment abnormality.
- Notching of the J point occurs with benign early repolarization.
- A positive deflection at the J point is termed a J wave (Osborn wave) and is characteristically seen with hypothermia.

ST SEGMENT

- The length between the end of the S wave (end of ventricular depolarization) and the beginning of repolarization **(Fig. 24)**

Chapter 4: Waves, Segments, and Intervals

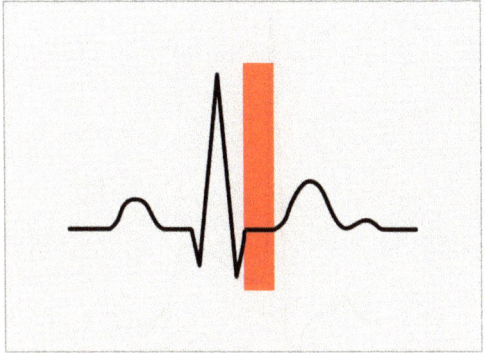

Fig. 24: ST segment.

- From J point on the end of QRS complex, to inclination of T wave
- Normally, all cells have the same potential = ST segment is electrically neutral (on isoelectric line)
- Ischemic focus has a different electric potential = electric vector leads to this area

1. **Subendocardial ischemia (non-Q-MI):** ST depression **(Fig. 25)**
2. **Subepicardial ischemia (Q-MI, aneurysm):** Elevation of ST segment **(Fig. 26)**

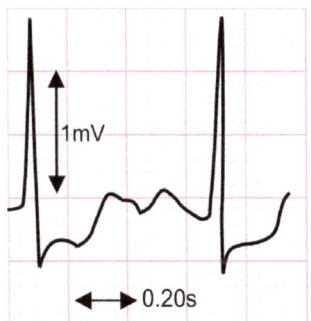

Fig. 25: Subendocardial ischemia—ST depression.

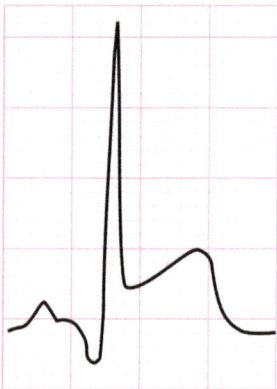

Fig. 26: Subepicardial ischemia—elevation of ST segment.

T WAVE

Normally: A repolarization directs from epicardium to endocardium = T wave is concordant with QRS complex.

It should be at least one tenth or 10% of the R wave amplitude in the same complex.

ST segment elevation (Fig. 27).

- Acute myocardial infarction
- Coronary vasospasm (Prinzmetal's angina)
- Pericarditis
- Early repolarization
- Pulmonary embolism
- Hypothermia
- Hypertrophic cardiomyopathy
- High potassium
- CVA
- Acute sympathetic stress
- Brugada syndrome.
- Cardiac aneurysm.
- Left ventricular hypertrophy
- Idioventricular rhythm including paced rhythm

Chapter 4: Waves, Segments, and Intervals

> **ST segment depression of 1 mm is found in many conditions (Fig. 28).**

- Ischemia
- Myocarditis
- Pericarditis
- Cardiomyopathy
- Pulmonary embolism
- Subarachnoid or cerebral hemorrhage
- Drugs: Digoxin effect, ethanol abuse
- Hyperventilation
- Electrolyte imbalance.

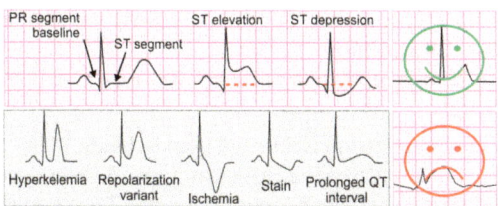

Fig. 27: ST segment deviations. The general rule of thumb is this: a "smiling" ST elevation is usually benign (pericarditis); a "frowning" ST elevation usually indicates imminent myocardial infarction.

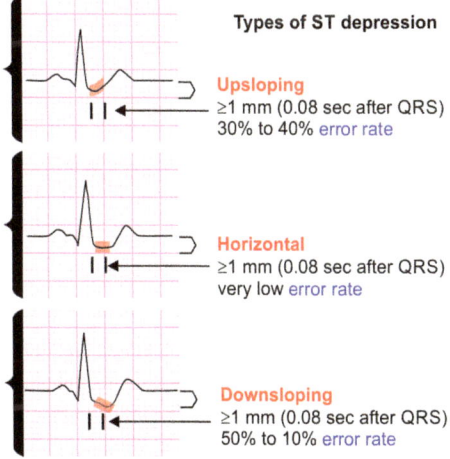

Fig. 28: Types of ST depression.

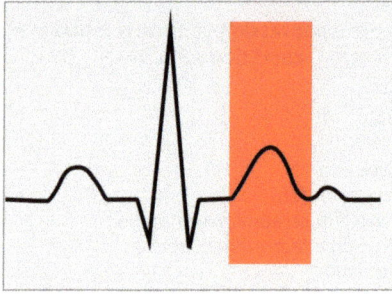

Fig. 29: Ventricular repolarization.

It is upright in leads I, II, aVF, and V2–V6 and inverted in aVR **(Figs. 29 and 30)**.

Ischemic area: A repolarization is delayed, an action potential is extended.

Vector of repolarization is directed from ischemic area:
- Subendocardial ischemia to epicardium—T wave elevation
- Subepicardial ischemia to endocardium—T wave inversion **(Fig. 31)**

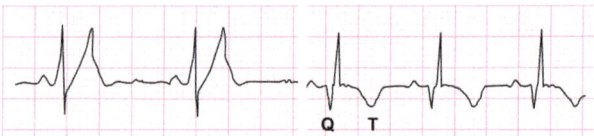

Fig. 31: Ischemic area—T wave elevation and inversion.

T wave inversions (Figs. 32 and 33).

- Myocardial ischemia
- LV overload
- Digitalis
- Pulmonary embolism
- Hypokalemia
- Pancreatitis, gallbladder disease
- Myocarditis/pericarditis
- Pneumothorax
- Cocaine/alcohol/caffeine
- Sympathetic overload—pheochromocytoma

Contd...

Chapter 4: Waves, Segments, and Intervals

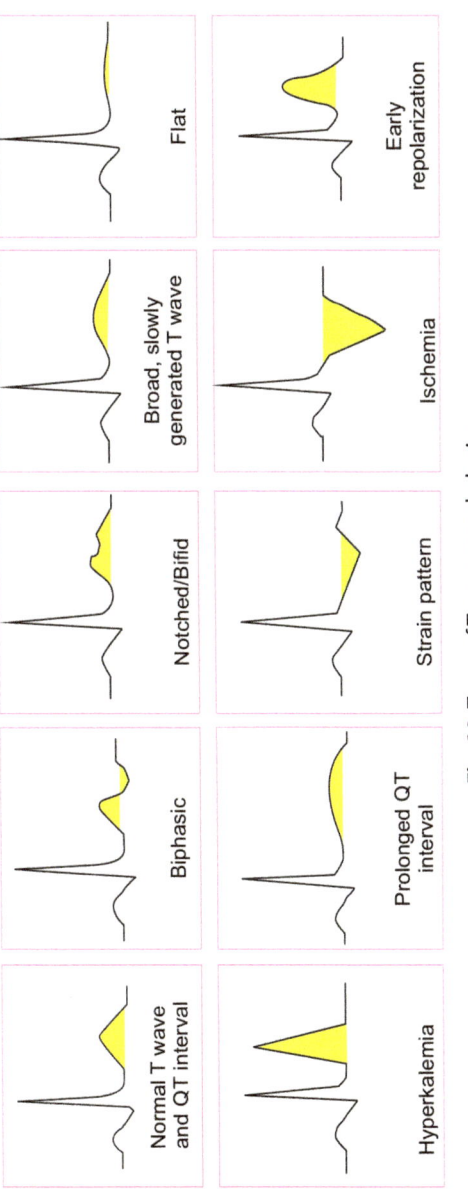

Fig. 30: Types of T wave morphologies.

Chapter 4: Waves, Segments, and Intervals

Contd...

- Ectopics and pacing
- Bundle branch blocks
- WPW syndrome
- Myxedema
- Idiopathic

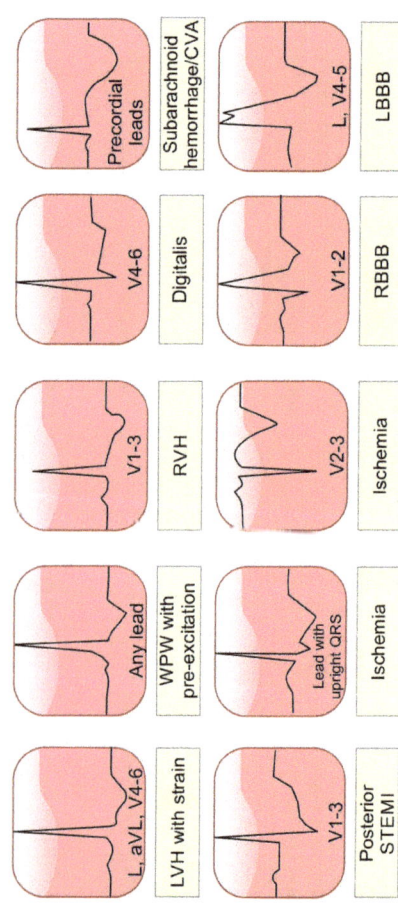

Fig. 32: Causes of ST depression and T wave inversion.

Chapter 4: Waves, Segments, and Intervals

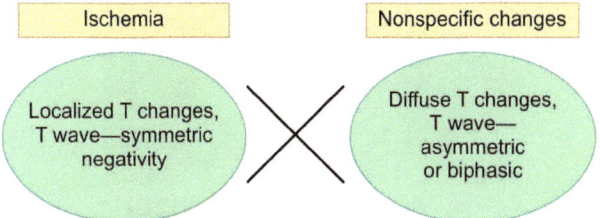

Fig. 33: Ischemic and nonspecific changes.

Deep T wave inversion of >5 mm (Fig. 34)
- CAD/ischemia
- HOCM- Apical
- SAH ("CVA -T wave pattern")
- Myocarditis, pericarditis

Tall T-waves:
When amplitude of T waves is >6 mm in limb leads or >10 mm in precordial leads OR height of T wave more than 2/3 of the neighboring QRS **(Fig. 35).**

Causes:
- Hyperacute T-waves—anterior wall MI
- Hyperkalemia
- True posterior wall MI (in V1, V2)
- BER
- LVH, BBB, pacing

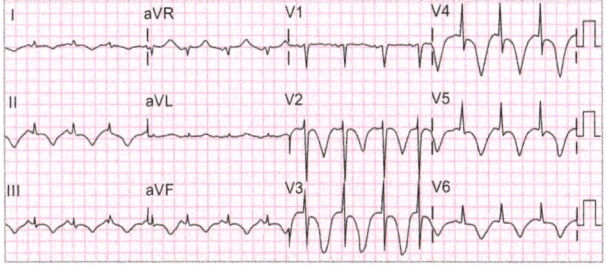

Fig. 34: Deep T wave inversion.

Chapter 4: Waves, Segments, and Intervals

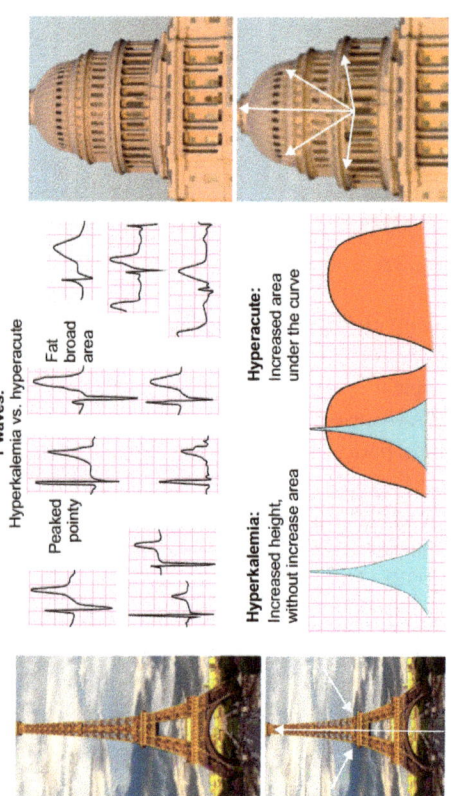

Fig. 35: Tall T waves.

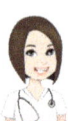

Nursing Considerations

- Assess specifically the potassium levels.
- Administer treatment as prescribed for hyperkalemia or hypokalemia.
- Monitor ABG of the patient if hemodynamically unstable or in critical settings like ICUs or HDUs.
- Monitor changes in ECG.

Chapter 4: Waves, Segments, and Intervals

QT-INTERVAL

Definition: Time interval between beginnings of QRS complex to the end of T wave.

Normally: At normal HR: QT ≤11 mm (0.44 sec).

Abnormalities:
1. *Prolonged QT interval:* Hypocalcemia and congenital long QT syndrome.
2. *Short QT interval:* Hypercalcemia.
   - The QT shortens at faster heart rates
   - The QT lengthens at slower heart rates.
   - An abnormally prolonged QT is associated with an increased risk of ventricular arrhythmias, especially Torsades de Pointes.
   - Congenital short QT syndrome has been found to be associated with an increased risk of paroxysmal atrial and ventricular fibrillation and sudden cardiac death.

QT interval decreases when heart rate increases.

A general guide to the upper limit of QT interval. For HR = 70 bpm, QT <0.40 sec.

- For every 10 bpm increase above 70 subtract 0.02 seconds.
- For every 10 bpm decrease below 70 add 0.02 seconds.

As a general guide the QT interval should be 0.35–0.45 seconds (<2 large square) and should not be more than half of the interval between adjacent R waves (R-R interval) **(Fig. 36)**.

Calculation of QT interval

- Use lead II. Use lead V5 alternatively, if lead II cannot be read.
- Draw a line through the baseline (preferably the PR segment).
- Draw a tangent against the steepest part of the end of the T wave. If the T wave has two positive deflections, the taller deflection should be chosen. If the T wave is biphasic, the end of the taller deflection should be chosen.
- The QT interval starts at the beginning of the QRS interval and ends where the tangent and baseline cross.
- If the QRS duration exceeds 120 ms the amount surpassing, 120 ms should be deducted from the QT interval [i.e., QT = QT − (QRS width − 120 ms)].

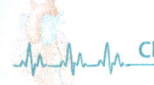

Chapter 4: Waves, Segments, and Intervals

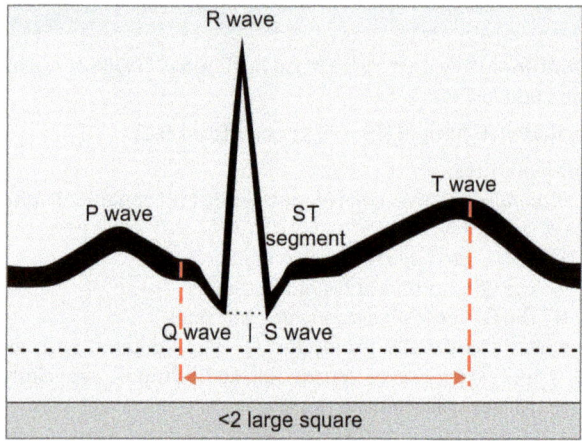

Fig. 36: QT-interval.

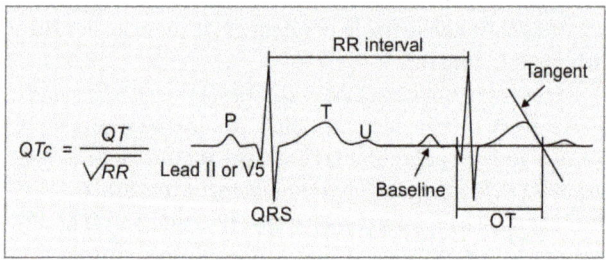

Fig. 37: QTc. Bazett's formula.

- To calculate the heart rate-corrected QT interval.
- *QTc*. **Bazett's formula** is used **(Fig. 37)**.

If abnormally prolonged or shortened, there is a risk of developing ventricular arrhythmias.

The QT interval is prolonged in congenital long QT syndrome, but QT prolongation can also occur as a consequence of:
- Medication (anti-arrhythmics, tricyclic antidepressants, and phenothiazines)
- Electrolyte imbalances
- Ischemia.

Long QT syndrome

Long QT is a rare inborn heart condition in which repolarization of the heart is delayed following a heartbeat **(Fig. 38)**.

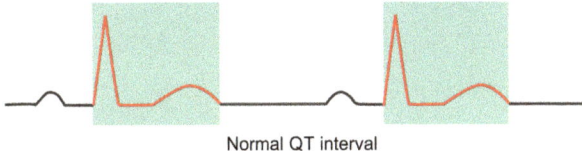

Normal QT interval

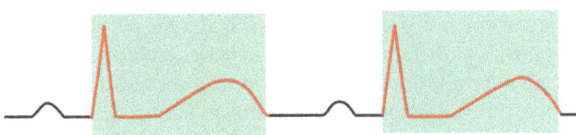

Prolonged or abnormal QT interval

Fig. 38: Long QT interval.

Example: Jervell and Lange–Nielsen syndrome or Romano–Ward syndrome

U WAVE

It is typically small, and by definition, follows the T wave. U waves are thought to represent repolarization of the papillary muscles or Purkinje fibers **(Fig. 39)**.

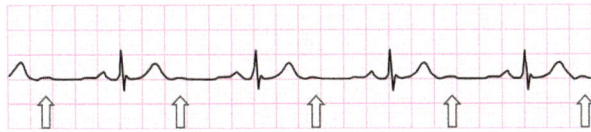

Fig. 39: U wave.

Prominent U waves are most often seen in **hypokalemia**, but may be present in hypercalcemia, thyrotoxicosis, or exposure to digitalis, epinephrine, and Class 1A and 3 antiarrhythmics, as well as in congenital long QT syndrome, thyrotoxicosis, and in the setting of intracranial hemorrhage.

An inverted-U wave may represent myocardial ischemia (may be the earliest sign) or left ventricular volume overload.

ECG in Myocardial Infarction

ACUTE CORONARY SYNDROME

An acute coronary syndrome (ACS) may include various clinical entities that involve some sort of ischemia or infarction. Specifically, acute coronary syndrome includes unstable angina, non-ST-segment elevation myocardial infarction (NSTEMI), and ST-segment elevation myocardial infarction (STEMI). Occasionally, NSTEMI is referred to as non-Q wave myocardial infarction and STEMI is referred to as Q wave myocardial infarction **(Fig. 1)**. This is because STEMI is almost always associated with a pathological Q wave.

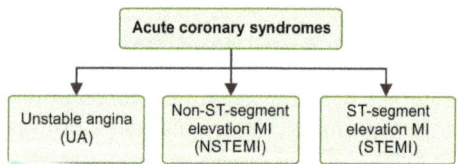

Fig. 1: Types of an acute coronary syndrome.
(MI: myocardial infarction)

MYOCARDIAL INFARCTION

For the patients to be diagnosed with myocardial infarction, they must have at least two of the following three criteria, according to the World Health Organization (WHO):
1. Clinical history of chest discomfort consistent with ischemia such as crushing chest pain
2. An elevation of cardiac markers in the blood (troponin-I, CK-MB, myoglobin)
3. Characteristic changes on electrocardiographic tracings taken serially

Chapter 5: ECG in Myocardial Infarction

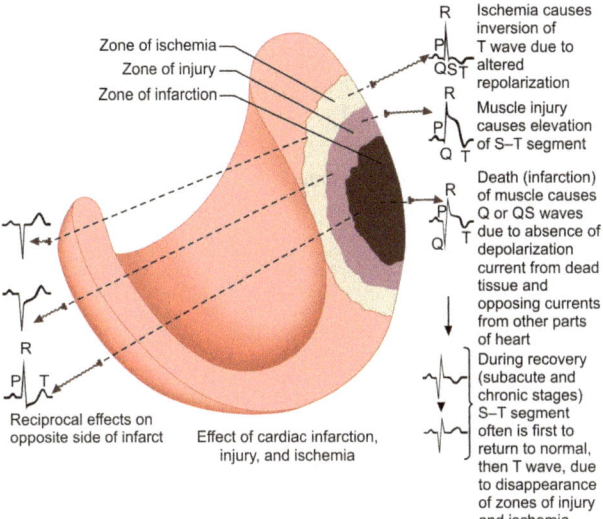

Fig. 2: ECG changes due to MI.

Recognition of infarction on the ECG relies on the detection of morphologic changes (i.e., changes in shape) of the QRS complex, the T-wave, and the ST-segment. These changes occur in relation to certain events during the infarction.

Figure 2 shows the ECG changes due to STEMI that often occur in a predictable pattern. The ECG changes appear only in leads looking at the infarct site. These changes are referred to as the indicative changes of myocardial infarction.

ECG Changes: Ischemia (Fig. 3)

- T-wave inversion (flipped T)
- ST-segment depression
- T-wave flattening
- Biphasic T-waves

ECG Changes: Injury

- ST-segment elevation of >1 mm in at least 2 contiguous leads **(Fig. 4)**

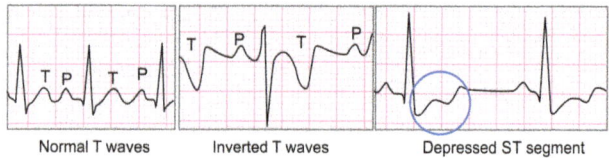

Fig. 3: ECG changes in ischemia.

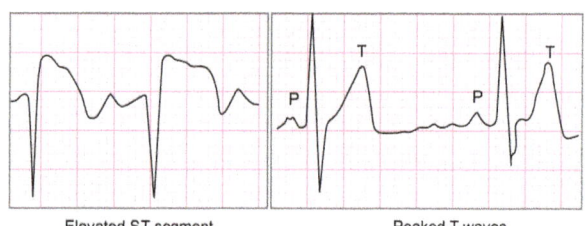

Fig. 4: ECG changes in injury.

- Heightened or peaked T-waves
- Directly related to portions of myocardium rendered electrically inactive

What is significant St elevation?

The important recommendations for significant ST elevation are given in **Box 1** and described in **Figures 5A to D**.

Box 1: Recommendations for significant ST elevation.

1. For men 40 years of age and older, the threshold value for abnormal J-point elevation should be 0.2 mV (2 mm) in leads V2 and V3 and 0.1 mV (1 mm) in all other leads.
2. For men less than 40 years of age, the threshold values for abnormal J-point elevation in leads V2 and V3 should be 0.25 mV (2.5 mm).
3. For women, the threshold value for abnormal J-point elevation should be 0.15 mV (1.5 mm) in leads V2 and V3 and greater than 0.1 mV (1 mm) in all other leads.

Contd...

Contd...

4. For men and women, the threshold for abnormal J-point elevation in V3R and V4R should be 0.05 mV (0.5 mm), except for males less than 30 years of age, for whom 0.1 mV (1 mm) is more appropriate.
5. For men and women, the threshold value for abnormal J-point elevation in V7 through V9 should be 0.05 mV (0.5 mm).
6. For men and women of all ages, the threshold value for abnormal J-point depression should be -0.05 mV (-0.5 mm) in leads V2 and V3 and -0.1 mV (-1 mm) in all other leads.

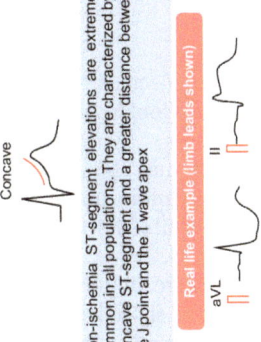

Characteristics of ST-segment elevations caused by ischemia

Convex | Straight upsloping | Straight horizontal | Straight downsloping

A: ST-segment elevations caused by ischemia typically displays a convex or straight ST-segment. Such ST-segment elevations in presence of chest discomfort are strongly suggestive of transmural myocardial ischemia. Note that the straight downsloping variant is unusual

Examples of ST-segment elevations caused by ischemia

C: ST-segment elevation can vary markedly in appearance. These six examples were retrieved from six different patients with STEMI

Typical non-ischemic ST-segment elevation

Concave

B: Non-ischemia ST-segment elevations are extremely common in all populations. They are characterized by a concave ST-segment and a greater distance between the J point and the T wave apex

Real life example (limb leads shown)

aVL | I | -aVR
II | aVF | III

D: ECG from a make patient (age 61) who experienced chest pain while driving to work. Note ST-segment elevations as well as reciprocal ST-segment depressions. There are also pathological Q-waves (leads III, aVF and perhaps II)

Figs. 5A to D: Significant ST elevation.

Chapter 5: ECG in Myocardial Infarction

ECG Changes: Infarct

- Significant Q wave where none previously existed
- Impulse traveling away from the positive lead
- Necrotic tissue is electrically dead
- Criteria:
  - Depth of Q wave should be 25% the height of the R wave
  - Width of Q wave is 0.04 s
  - Diminished height of the R wave

Evolving MI and Hallmarks of AMI

Figures 6A to E shows pattern of changes in evolving AMI.

Reciprocal Changes

- ECG signs of myocardial injury are reflected by the presence of ST-segment *elevation* in the leads looking directly at the affected area.
- The uninvolved areas of the heart may show ST-segment *depression*. This is called a reciprocal ("mirror image") change.
- Reciprocal changes are seen in the wall of the heart opposite the location of the infarction **(Fig. 7)**.
- Reciprocal changes are usually most readily observed at the onset of an infarction and tend to be short lived.
- When present, reciprocal changes strongly suggest an acute infarction.
- Reciprocal changes are seen in approximately 75% of inferior wall MIs and approximately 30% of anterior wall MIs.

LOCALIZATION OF MI BASED ON ECG

Location of MI	Leads affected	Vessel involved	ECG changes
Anterior wall	V2 to V4	Left anterior descending artery (LAD)—diagonal branch	• Poor R-wave progression • ST-segment elevation • T-wave inversion

Contd...

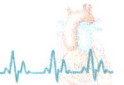

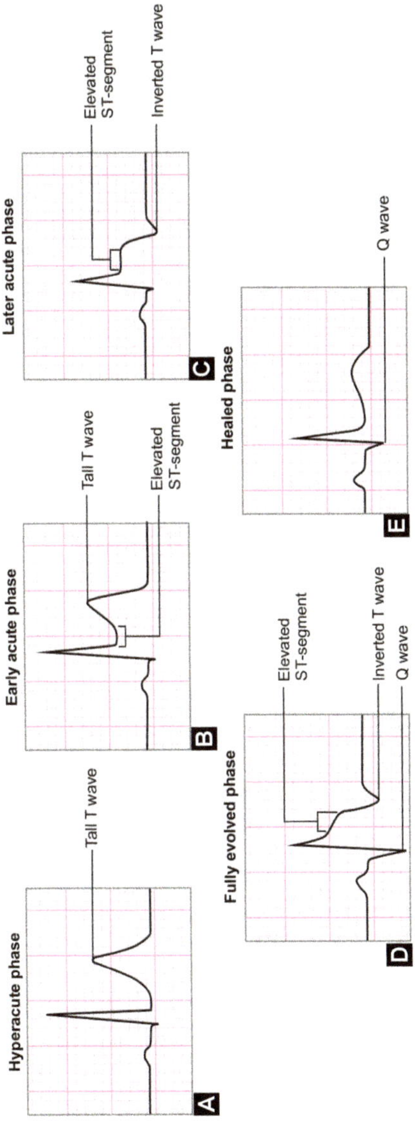

Figs. 6A to E: Pattern of changes in evolving AMI.

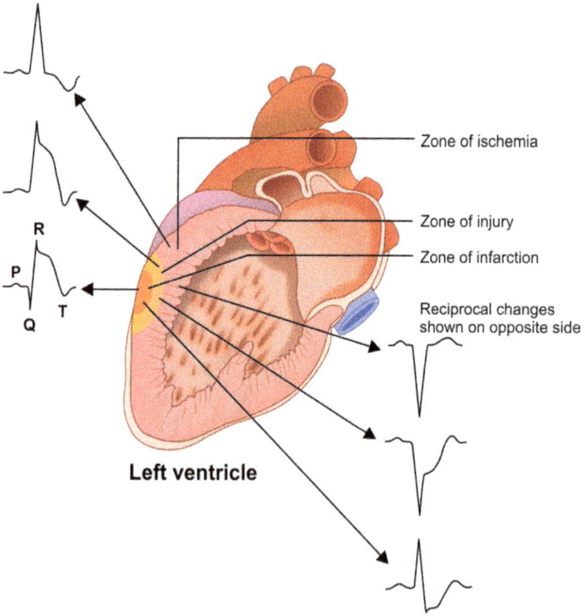

Chapter 5: ECG in Myocardial Infarction

Fig. 7: Reciprocal changes are seen in the wall of the heart.

Contd...

Location of MI	Leads affected	Vessel involved	ECG changes
Septal wall	V1 and V2	Left anterior descending artery (LAD)—septal branch	• R-wave disappears • ST-segment rises • T-wave inverts
Lateral wall	I, aVL, V5, V6	Left aoronary artery (LCA)—circumflex branch	• ST-segment elevation
Inferior wall	II, III, aVF	Right coronary artery (RCA)—Posterior descending branch	• T-wave inversion • ST-segment elevation

Contd...

Chapter 5: ECG in Myocardial Infarction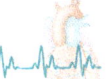

Contd...

Location of MI	Leads affected	Vessel involved	ECG changes
Posterior wall	V1 to V4	• Left coronary artery (LCA)—circumflex branch • Right coronary artery (RCA)—Posterior descending branch	• Tall R-waves • ST-segment depression • Upright T-waves

NON-ST ELEVATION MYOCARDIAL INFARCTION

NSTEMI is diagnosed in patients who have symptoms consistent with acute coronary syndrome (ACS) and troponin elevation, but without ECG changes consistent with STEMI.

ECG Manifestation

- ST depressions and T-wave inversions
- ST depression can be either upsloping, downsloping or horizontal **(Fig. 8)**
- Horizontal or downsloping ST depression ≥0.5 mm at the J-point in ≥2 contiguous leads indicates myocardial ischemia
- ST depression ≥ 1 mm is more specific and conveys a worse prognosis
- ST depression ≥2 mm in ≥3 leads is associated with a high probability of NSTEMI and predicts significant mortality (6 x higher risk of death)
- Upsloping ST depression is nonspecific for myocardial ischemia.
- Presence of widespread ST depressions plus ST elevation in aVR >1 mm is suggestive of left main coronary artery occlusion

T-wave inversion must fulfill these criteria:

- Be present in ≥2 contiguous leads that have dominant R-waves (R/S ratio >1)
- Be dynamic
- Be at least 1 mm deep

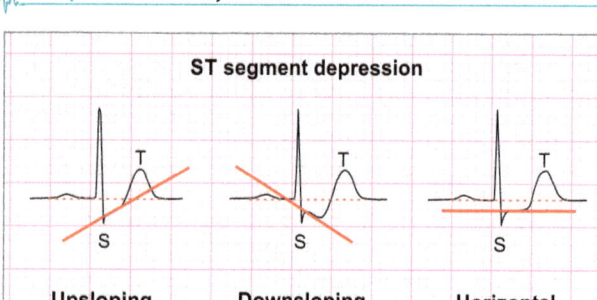

Fig. 8: ST segment depression.

COMPLICATIONS OF ACUTE CORONARY SYNDROME

The complications of ACS are given in Table 1.

Table 1: Complications of acute coronary syndrome.	
Type	*Manifestation*
Ischemic	Reinfarction
	Infarct extension
	Angina
Mechanical	Cardiac failure
	Cardiogenic shock
	Mitral regurgitation
	Ventricular aneurysm
	Cardiac rupture (ventricular septum, papillary muscle or cardiac wall)
Arrhythmic	Atrial or ventricular arrhythmia
	Sinus or atrioventricular node dysfunction
Embolic	Central nervous system embolus (especially stroke)
	Peripheral embolus
	Left ventricular mural thrombus
Inflammatory	Pericarditis

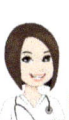

Nursing Considerations

- Strict bed rest.
- Obtain ECG daily.
- Ensure patent IV access with large bore catheters.
- Monitor cardiac enzymes.
- Administer morphine as prescribed.
- Administer aspirin and nitroglycerin (0.4 mg sublingual) as ordered.
- Provide oxygen therapy.
- Monitor vital signs, daily weight, and urine output.
- Administer heparin as prescribed for STEMI.
- Educate the patient to eat healthy and low salt diet, medication compliance, controlling blood pressure, blood sugars and lipids, and maintaining body weight.

Tachyarrhythmia

CHAPTER 6

INTRODUCTION

Tachydysrhythmias are defined as any abnormal cardiac rhythm with a rate greater than 100 beats per minute.

A systematic approach can be useful in the rapid assessment and treatment of the patient presenting with tachydysrhythmia.

It is important to recognize the hemodynamic consequences of the rhythm. General approach to tachyarrhythmias are shown in **Flowchart 1**.

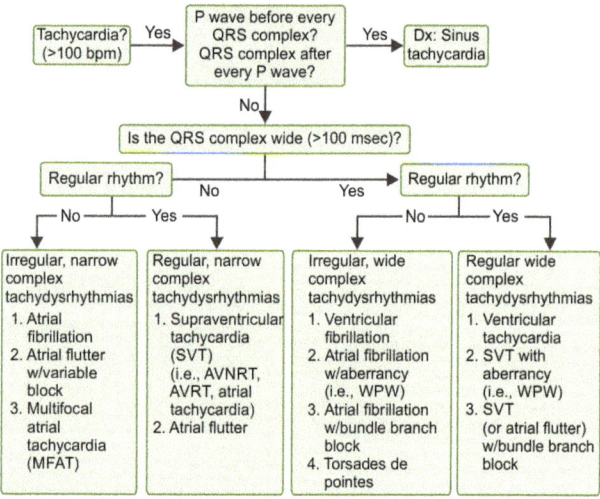

Flowchart 1: General approach to tachyarrhythmias.

Narrow QRS complex

Regular
- Supraventricular tachycardia (SVT)
- Sinus tachycardia
- Atrial flutter
- Junctional rhythm

Irregular
- Atrial fibrillation
- Atrial flutter with variable block
- Multifocal atrial tachycardia

Wide QRS complex

Regular
- Ventricular tachycardia
- SVT with aberrancy

Irregular
- Atrial fibrillation with pre-excitation
- AF with aberrancy
- Ventricular fibrillation
- Torsades de pointes

NARROW COMPLEX TACHYDYSRHYTHMIAS

Sinus Rhythm

It occurs when the electrical impulse starts at a regular rate and rhythm in the sinus node and travels through the normal conduction pathway (**Fig. 1**).

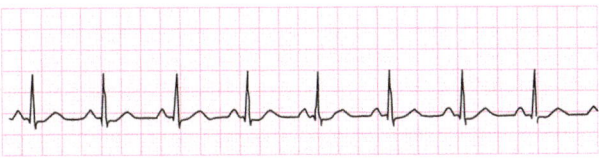

Fig. 1: Electrocardiogram showing sinus rhythm.

ECG Characteristics

Ventricular and atrial rate	60–100 bpm
Ventricular and atrial rhythm	Regular
QRS complex	Normal
P wave	Normal and consistent shape
PR interval	Consistent interval between 0.12–0.20 second.

Sinus Tachycardia

It occurs when the sinus node creates an impulse at a faster-than-normal.

Sinus tachycardia (ST) is the most common narrow complex regular tachycardia. ST is characterized by sinus P waves, normal PR interval (<200 msec), 1:1 AV conduction, and an atrial rate usually 100–160 beats/min. It is typically an appropriate response to physiologic stimuli. Common causes include: hypovolemia, sepsis, pain, alcohol withdrawal, sympathomimetic intoxication, thyroid storm, etc. (**Figs. 2 and 3**).

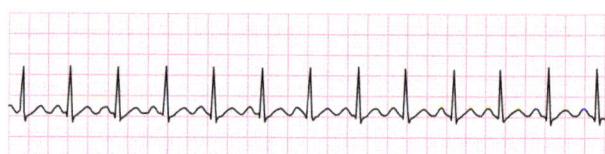

Fig. 2: Electrocardiogram showing sinus tachycardia.

ECG Characteristics

Ventricular and atrial rate	>100 to <120 bpm
Ventricular and atrial rhythm	Regular
QRS complex	Usually normal but may be regularly abnormal
P wave	Normal and consistent shape
PR interval	Consistent interval between 0.12 and 0.20 seconds

Chapter 6: Tachyarrhythmia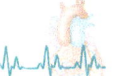

Medical Management
- ❖ Administration of beta blockers and calcium channel blockers.
- ❖ Catheter ablation of SA node.

Nursing Considerations

- Assess the heart rate periodically.
- Reassure the patient.
- Encourage the fluid and sodium intake.
- Assess for adequate cardiac output and notify the provider if indicated.
- Educate about lifestyle changes.

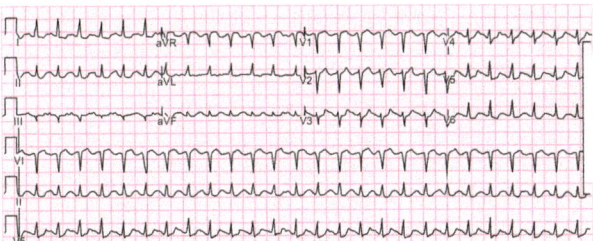

Fig. 3: Electrocardiogram showing sinus tachycardia with different features.

It is a normal phenomenon that occurs with changes in intrathoracic pressure. The heart rate increase with inspiration (RR interval shorten) and decreases with expiration (RR interval lengthen), so the rhythm is irregular.

Loss of sinus arrhythmia is seen in seen in cardiac failure and autonomic neuropathy.

Atrial Flutter

It occurs because of a conduction defect in the atrium and causes a rapid, regular atrial rate, usually between 250 to 400 times per minute. Because the atrial rate is faster than the AV node can conduct, not all atrial impulses are conducted into the ventricle, causing a therapeutic block at the AV node.

Chapter 6: Tachyarrhythmia

These are the important features.
- Narrow complex tachycardia
- Regular atrial activity at approximately 300 bpm
- Flutter waves ("saw-tooth" pattern) best seen in leads II, III, aVF—may be more easily spotted by turning the ECG upside down **(Fig. 4)**
- Flutter waves in V1 may resemble P waves
- Loss of the isoelectric baseline.

Signs and Symptoms

Chest pain, shortness of breath, and low blood pressure.

Causes

Chronic obstructive pulmonary disease (COPD), valvular disease, and thyrotoxicosis, as well as following open heart surgery and repair of congenital cardiac defect.

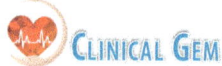

Signs and symptoms depend on ventricular response rate.

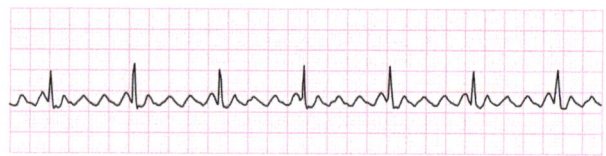

Fig. 4: Atrial flutter.

ECG Characteristics

Atrial rate	Ranges between 250–400 bpm
Ventricular rate	Usually ranges between 75–150 bpm
Ventricular and atrial rhythm	The atrial rhythm is regular; the ventricular rhythm is usually regular but may be irregular because of a change in the AV conduction

Contd...

Contd...

QRS complex	Usually normal but may be abnormal or may be absent
P wave	Saw-toothed shape; these waves are referred to as F waves
PR interval	Multiple F waves may make it difficult to determine the PR interval

Medical Management

- Vagal maneuvers or administration of adenosine intravenously, followed by a 20-mL saline flush and elevation of the arm with the IV line to promote rapid circulation of the medication.
- Electrical cardioversion
- Medications used to slow the ventricular response rate include beta-blockers, non-dihydropyridine calcium channel blockers and digitalis.
- Catheter ablation.

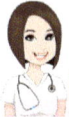

Nursing Considerations

- Carefully observe the atrial and ventricular rates.
- Monitor for signs of decreased cardiac output and stroke.

Supraventricular Tachycardia

- Refer to any tachydysrhythmia arising from above the level of the bundle of His.
- Paroxysmal SVT (pSVT) describes an SVT with abrupt onset and offset—characteristically seen with re-entrant tachycardias involving the AV node such as AVNRT or atrioventricular re-entry tachycardia (AVRT) **(Figs. 5 and 6)**.

Chapter 6: Tachyarrhythmia

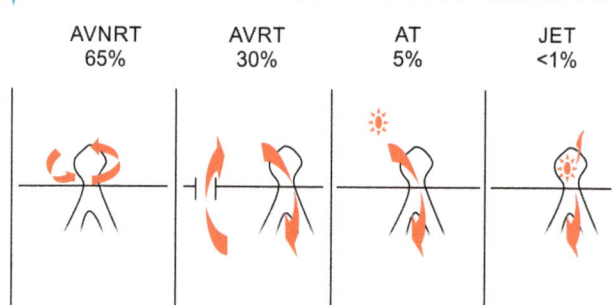

Fig. 5: Mechanism of pSVT.

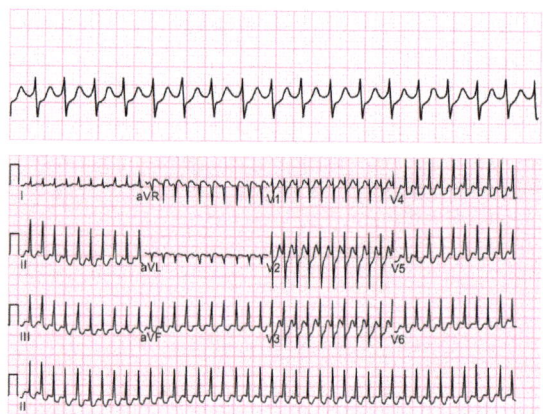

Fig. 6: Electrocardiogram showing supraventricular tachycardia.

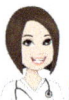

Nursing Considerations

- Administer oxygen with nasal cannula as ordered.
- Monitor ECG and vital signs and notify the abnormality to the physician.
- Assist with cardioversion.
- Administer the medications as ordered.
- Assess vital signs, level of consciousness, level of sedation, capillary refill, cardiovascular, and respiratory status following cardioversion.

Clinical Gems

- SVT can be related to caffeine intake, nicotine, stress, or anxiety in healthy adults.
- Patients may experience angina, hypotension, light-headedness, palpitations, and intense anxiety.

Atrial Fibrillation

- It is the most common sustained arrhythmia.
- It is an uncoordinated atrial electrical activation that causes a rapid, disorganized, and uncoordinated twitching of atrial musculature.
- The incidence and prevalence of AF is increasing.
- Lifetime risk over the age of 40 years is ~25% **(Fig. 7)**.

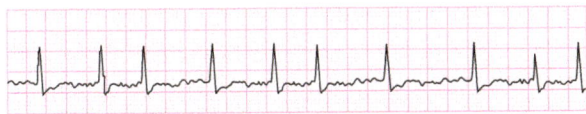

Fig. 7: Atrial fibrillation.

- **Irregularly irregular rhythm.**
- **No P waves**. Atrial rate: 600
- Absence of an isoelectric baseline.
- Variable ventricular rate.
- QRS complexes usually <120 ms unless pre-existing bundle branch block, accessory pathway, or rate related aberrant conduction.
- **Fibrillary waves** may be present and can be either fine (amplitude <0.5 mm) or coarse (amplitude >0.5 mm).
- AF is often described as having "**rapid ventricular response**" once the ventricular rate is >100 bpm **(Fig. 8)**.
- "**Slow**" **AF** is a term often used to describe AF with a ventricular rate <60 bpm.
  - Causes of "slow" AF include hypothermia, digoxin toxicity, medications, and sinus node dysfunction.

Chapter 6: Tachyarrhythmia

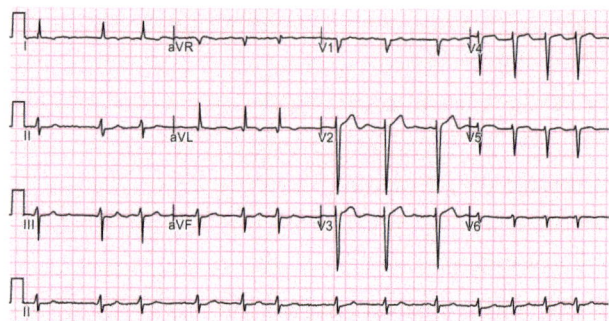

Fig. 8: Atrial fibrillation with a controlled ventricular rate.

Etiology of Atrial Fibrillation

- Ischemic heart disease
- Hypertension
- Valvular heart disease (especially mitral stenosis/regurgitation)
- Acute infections
- Electrolyte disturbance (hypokalemia, hypomagnesemia)
- Thyrotoxicosis
- Drugs (e.g., sympathomimetics)
- Pulmonary embolism
- Pericardial disease
- Acid-base disturbance
- Pre-excitation syndromes
- Cardiomyopathies: Dilated, hypertrophic.
- Pheochromocytoma

Treatment of AF

Treatment of AF has been described in **Flowchart 4**.

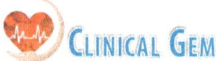

CLINICAL GEM

It is usually a chronic arrhythmia associated with underlying heart disease.

Chapter 6: Tachyarrhythmia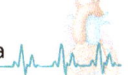

Flowchart 4: Treatment of AF.

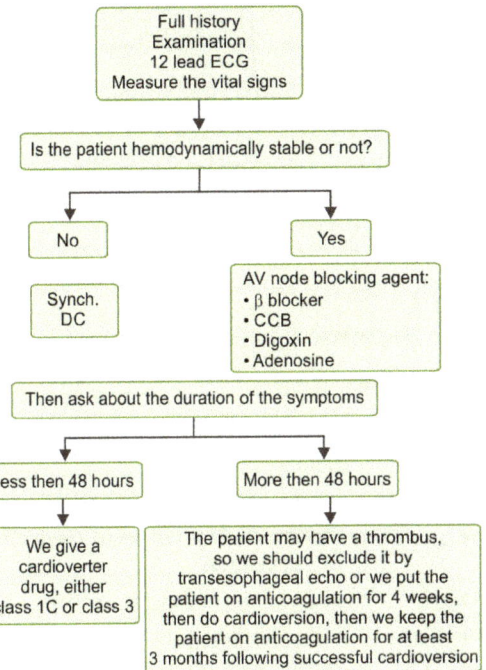

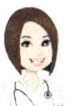

Nursing Considerations

- Obtain 12 lead ECG appearance: chaotic rhythm with no P waves
- Measure vitals—if unstable may need cardioversion
- Administer drugs as prescribed
- Administer anticoagulant
- Observe the neurological and cardiovascular status

Premature Ventricular Complex

A premature ventricular complex (PVC) is an impulse that starts in a ventricle and is conducted through the ventricles before the next normal sinus impulse **(Fig. 9)**.

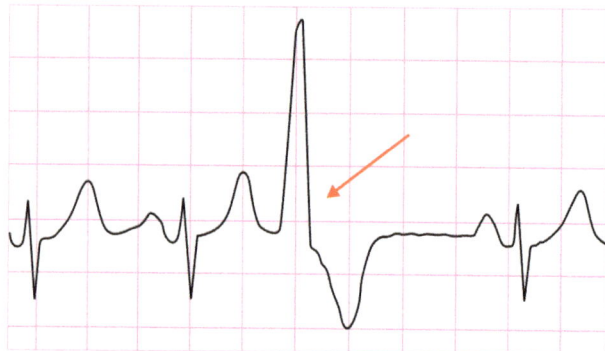

Fig. 9: Premature ventricular complex.

ECG Characteristics

Rhythm	Irregular
Atrial rate	Normal
Ventricular rate	Normal
P-wave	Absent with PVC, but present with other QRS complexes
PR interval	0.12 sec with underlying rhythm
QRS complex	Early with bizarre configuration
T-wave	Normal; opposite direction with QRS complex with PVC
Other	Compensatory pause after PVC

Causes

Electrolyte imbalances—hypokalemia, hyperkalemia, hypomagnesemia and hypocalcemia, metabolic acidosis, hypoxia, MI, ventricular hypertrophy, increased sympathetic stimulation, myocarditis, cardiomyopathy, HF, caffeine or alcohol ingestion, tobacco use.

Signs and Symptoms

Palpitations, hypotension, syncope, dyspnea, dizziness, decreased cardiac output evidenced by fatigue, decreased level of consciousness, cool peripheries, increased JVP, hypoxemia.

Medical Management

- Antiarrhythmics like lidocaine (first line), procaine or amiodarone
- Potassium chloride to correct hypokalemia, magnesium sulfate to correct hypomagnesemia, oxygen administration for hypoxia, radiofrequency catheter ablation, implantable cardioverter defibrillator.

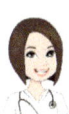

Nursing Considerations

- Patients who have recently developed PVCs need prompt assessment, especially if they have underlying heart disease or complex medical problems.
- Frequently stressed individuals should consider therapy or joining a support group.
- Those with chronic PVCs should be observed closely for the development of more frequent PVCs or more dangerous PVC patterns.
- Until an effective treatment is begun, patients with PVCs accompanied by serious symptoms should have continuous ECG monitoring and ambulate only with assistance.
- If the patient is discharged from healthcare facility on antiarrhythmic drugs, family members should know—how to contract the emergency medical service and how to perform cardiopulmonary resuscitation (CPR).

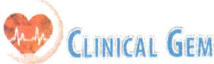

Patients may sense PVCs as skipped beats. Because the ventricles are only partially filled, the PVC frequently does not generate a pulse.

Idioventricular Rhythm

It is also termed as ventricular escape rhythm. It occurs when the impulse starts in the conduction system below the AV node.

Chapter 6: Tachyarrhythmia

When the sinus node fails to create an impulse, or when the impulse is created but cannot be conducted through the AV node, the Purkinje fibers automatically discharge an impulse. (**Fig. 10**)

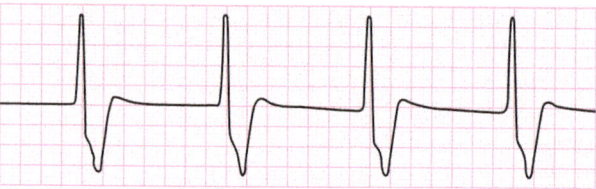

Fig. 10: Idioventricular rhythm.

ECG Characteristics

Rhythm	Atrial rhythm cannot be determined. Ventricular rhythm is regular
Atrial rate	Cannot be determined
Ventricular rate	20-40 bpm
P-wave	Absent
PR interval	Cannot measure
QRS complex	Longer than 0.12 sec with a wide and bizarre configuration
T-wave	Deflection opposite to the direction of QRS complex (discordance)
QT interval	Prolonged

Causes

May accompany third degree heart blocks or caused by myocardial ischemia or infraction, digoxin toxicity, beta-adrenergic blockers, pacemaker failure, metabolic imbalances.

Signs and Symptoms

Earlier patients may have—palpitations, dizziness, light-headedness, syncope. If the arrhythmias persist patients may have hypotension, weak peripheral pulses, decreased urine output, confusion.

Medical Management

- Atropine may be prescribed to increase the heart rate.
- Pacemaker

Chapter 6: Tachyarrhythmia

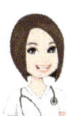

Nursing Considerations

- Patient needs constant assessment and continuous ECG monitoring until treatment restores hemodynamic stability.
- If a permanent pacemaker is inserted, teach the patient and his family how it works, how to recognize problems, when to contact the healthcare workers and how to monitor pacemaker function.

Ventricular Tachycardia (VT)

VT is defined as three or more PVCs in a row, occurring at a rate exceeding 100 bpm **(Figs. 11 and 12)**.

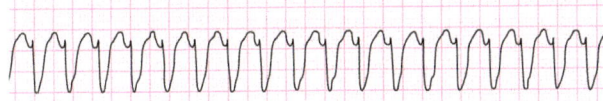

Fig. 11: Electrocardiogram showing ventricular tachycardia.

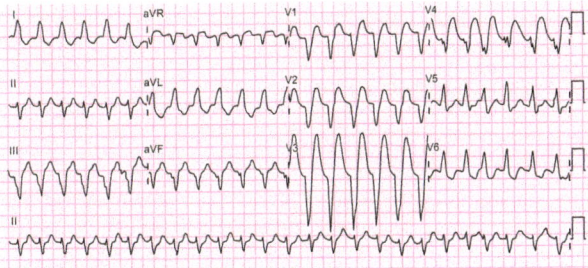

Fig. 12: Ventricular tachycardia.

ECG Characteristics

Rhythm	Generally regular but may be sightly irregular
Atrial rate	Depends on the underlying rhythm
Ventricular rate	100–220 bpm
P-wave	Very difficult to detect
PR interval	Very irregular if P-wave is seen
QRS complex	Broad and bizarre, duration is 0.12 seconds
T-wave	Cannot be determined
QT interval	Cannot be determined

Causes

Acute MI, coronary artery disease, SLE, myocarditis, heart failure, RA, chronic ischemic heart disease, electrolyte imbalances—hypokalemia and hypomagnesemia, cardiomyopathy, digitalis toxicity, ventricular aneurysm, heart surgery, previous damage to the heart.

Signs and Symptoms

Chest pain, lightheadedness, shortness of breath, increased JVP, palpitations, anxiety, syncope, hypotension, tachypnea, decreased LOC.

A. Monomorphic VT

In monomorphic VT, the QRS complexes have the same shape and amplitude **(Fig. 13)**.

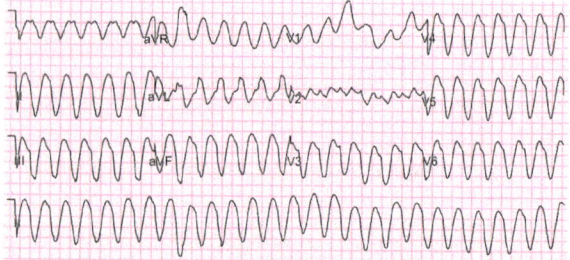

Fig. 13: Monomorphic VT.

ECG Characteristics

Rate	100–250 bpm
Rhythm	Regular
P-waves	None
PR interval	None
QRS	Wide (>0.10 sec), bizarre appearance

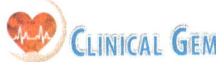

CLINICAL GEM

If left untreated, monomorphic VT will likely progress into VF or unstable VT.

B. Polymorphic VT

In polymorphic VT, QRS complexes are varied shape and amplitude **(Fig. 14)**.

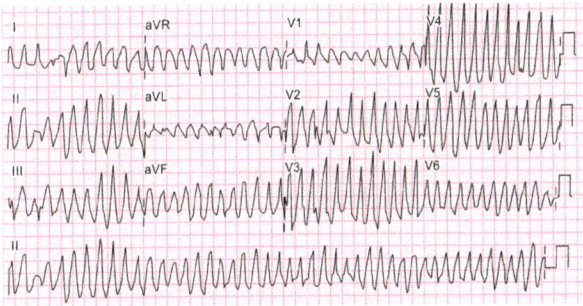

Fig. 14: Polymorphic VT.

ECG Characteristics

Rate	100–250 bpm
Rhythm	Regular or irregular
P-waves	None
PR interval	None
QRS	Wide (>0.10 sec), bizarre appearance

Chapter 6: Tachyarrhythmia

Medical Management

It is a medical emergency—defibrillation, cardioversion, implantable ICD, catheter ablation. For those who are stable with a monomorphic waveform the anti-arrhythmic medications can be used.

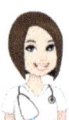

Nursing Considerations

- Assessing the condition of a patient.
- Differentiate between VT with pulse or without pulse.
- If the pulse is present:
  - Provide oxygen.
- Ensure patent IV access.
- Monitor the patient very closely.
- If pulseless
  - Activate code blue.
  - Begin CPR
  - Defibrillate at the earliest.
  - Start IV if not already established.
  - Notify the on-duty physician.
  - Treat reversible causes appropriately (5Ts and 5Hs)

Torsades de Pointes

Torsade de pointes is a polymorphic VT preceded by a prolonged QT interval **(Fig. 15)**.

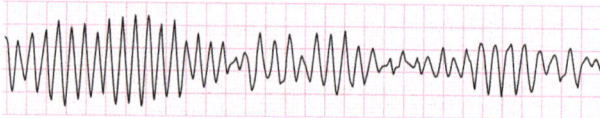

Fig. 15: Electrocardiogram showing Torsades de pointes.

Rate	V: 150–200
Rhythm	Irregular
QRS	QRS complexes display "spindle-node" pattern
Feature	No recognizable P and T waves, prolong QT before occurrence

Contd...

Contd...

- Torsades de pointes is associated with QTc prolongation, which is the heart rate adjusted lengthening of the QT interval
- Acquired QTc prolongation is most often drug-related (antiarrhythmics, antipsychotics, antiemetics, antifungals, and antimicrobials)
- Congenital prolonged QT has two genetic variants: Jervell and Lange–Nielsen and Romano–Ward syndrome
- Pulseless Torsades should be defibrillated. Intravenous magnesium is the first-line pharmacologic therapy in Torsades de pointes.

Clinical Gem

It can deteriorate to VF or asystole.

Ventricular Fibrillation

It is the most common dysrhythmia in patients with cardiac arrest. It is a rapid, disorganized ventricular rhythm that causes ineffective quivering of the ventricles **Figure 16**.

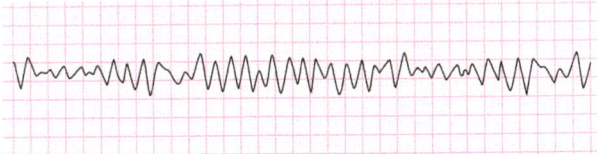

Fig. 16: Electrocardiogram showing ventricular fibrillation.

ECG Characteristics

Rhythm	Extremely irregular (Chaotic)
Atrial rate	Cannot be determined
Ventricular rate	300-600 bpm
P-wave	Absent
PR interval	Cannot be determined
QRS complex	Fibrillatory baseline
T-wave	Cannot be determined
QT interval	Cannot be determined

Causes

Acute coronary syndrome, VT, electrolyte imbalances, metabolic acidosis.

Signs and Symptoms

Pulse disappears with onset of VF, collapse, unconsciousness, gasping.

Medical Management

- ❖ Oxygen therapy, defibrillation, CPR, intubation, follow AHA algorithm.

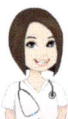

Nursing Considerations

- Activate code blue
- Provide CPR
- Administer medications as ordered.
- Draw blood sample for electrolytes, cardiac enzymes and toxicology screen.

Bradyarrhythmias

CHAPTER 7

SINUS BRADYCARDIA

It occurs when the sinus node creates an impulse at a slower-than-normal rate.

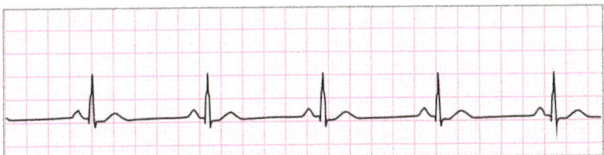

Fig. 1: Electrocardiogram showing sinus bradycardia.

ECG Characteristics

Rate	<60 beats/min
Rhythm	Regular sinus **(Fig. 1)**
PR	Regular; <0.20 seconds
P-waves	Size and shape normal; every P-wave is followed by a QRS complex; every QRS complex is preceded by a P-wave
QRS complex	Narrow; <0.10 seconds in absence of intraventricular conduction defect

Causes

Lower metabolic needs (e.g., sleep), vagal stimulation (e.g., vomiting, suctioning, severe pain), medications (e.g., calcium channel blockers, amiodarone, beta-blockers), increased intracranial pressure (ICP).

Medical Management

- Administer atropine
- Transcutaneous pacemaker

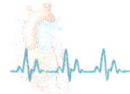

Chapter 7: Bradyarrhythmias

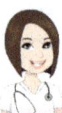

Nursing Considerations

- Assess the vital signs.
- Monitor the ECG.
- Administer Inj Atropine, 0.5 mg as an intravenous (IV) bolus every 3 to 5 minutes to a maximum total dose of 3 mg as ordered. It is the drug of choice in treating symptomatic sinus bradycardia.
- Assess for adequate cardiac output.
- Withhold cardiac medications if indicated and notify the physician.

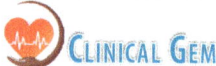

Sinus badycardia is normal in athletes and during sleep.

HEART BLOCK

- ❖ **Between the sinus node and atria**: SA block
- ❖ **Between the atria and ventricles:** AV block
- ❖ **Within the atria:** Intra-atrial block
- ❖ **Within the ventricles:** Intraventricular block

AV Block

It occurs when all the atrial impulses are conducted through the AV node into the ventricles at a rate slower than normal.

- ❖ **First degree AV block:**
  - ◆ PR interval >200 msec
  - ◆ Normal morphology and duration of the QRS complex and maintenance of 1:1 conduction **(Fig. 2)**
  - ◆ No dropped beat
- ❖ **Second degree AV block, Mobitz 1 (Wenckebach phenomenon):**
  - ◆ Progressive prolongation of PR intervals
  - ◆ PP intervals constant

Chapter 7: Bradyarrhythmias

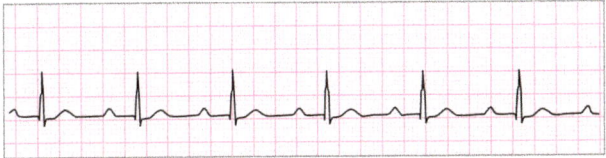

Fig. 2: Electrocardiogram showing first degree AV block.

- Dropped beat
  - PR interval is longest immediately before the dropped beat
  - PR interval is shortest immediately after the dropped beat
  - Constant PP interval and changing RR intervals with the cycle ending with a P wave not followed by a QRS complex **(Fig. 3)**

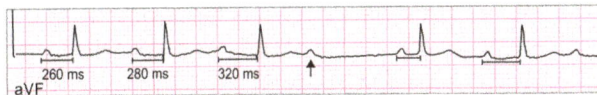

Fig. 3: Electrocardiogram showing second degree AV block Mobitz 1.

- The classic Wenckebach pattern occurs usually with ratios of 3:2, 4:3, or 5:4
- Occurs in up to 6% of healthy individuals

Second degree AV block, Mobitz II:
- Intermittent nonconducted P waves *without* progressive prolongation of the PR interval
- PR interval in the conducted beats remains constant
- *PP constant:* The P waves "march through" at a constant rate
- RR interval surrounding the dropped beat(s) is an exact multiple of the preceding RR interval
- In Mobitz type II, the block is generally located below the AV junction in the His bundle (intra-His block) or lower in the His-Purkinje system (infra-His block). Because of this, the QRS complexes are typically wide or demonstrate bundle branch block morphology **(Fig. 4)**

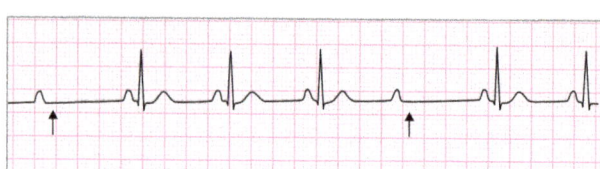

Fig. 4: Electrocardiogram showing second degree AV block Mobitz II.

- Mobitz II is much more likely than Mobitz I to be associated with hemodynamic compromise, severe bradycardia, and progression to third degree heart block—30% risk/year

❖ **Third degree AV block (complete heart block):**
  - Complete absence of AV conduction (AV dissociation): There is a complete interruption of conduction between atria and ventricles, so they work independently
  - The escape QRS rhythm is regular and originates in the junction or ventricles **(Fig. 5)**
    – Junctional escape rhythm with a narrow or wide QRS complex (supra-Hisian)
    – Ventricular escape rhythm with a wide QRS complex is more unreliable, slower

Although third-degree AV block is a form of AV dissociation (a condition in which atrial activation is independent from ventricular activation), not all AV dissociation represents third-degree AV block. Other causes could be, e.g., "interference-dissociation" due to the presence of a ventricular rhythm such as AIVR or VT.

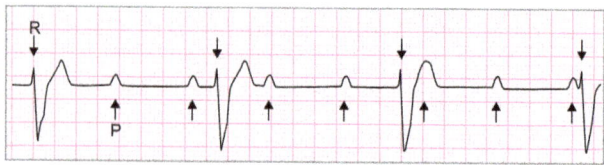

Fig. 5: Electrocardiogram showing third degree AV block.

> **Box 1:** Causes for AV block.

- **Myocardial infarction:** Anterior or inferior involving the conduction system
- **Drugs slowing down AV node conduction:** Digoxin, beta blockers, calcium channel blockers, many antiarrhythmic agents (propafenone, flecainide, procainamide, quinidine, and disopyramide)
- **Increased vagal tone (e.g., athletes):** Usually first degree and Wenckebach
- Idiopathic intrinsic degenerative diseases (Lenegre-Lev disease)
- **Myocarditis:** Lyme disease
- Infiltrative disease (sarcoidosis, amyloidosis)
- Hyperkalemia
- Autoimmune (SLE, systemic sclerosis)
- **Postcatheter ablation:** When in proximity to AV node
- Following transcatheter placement of valves
- Following cardiac surgery (mitral valve repair, TOF repair)

Sinus Node Dysfunction (SND)/Sick Sinus Syndrome

Sinus node dysfunction (SND) refers to a broad array of abnormalities in sinus node and atrial impulse formation and propagation. These include persistent sinus bradycardia and chronotropic incompetence without identifiable causes, paroxysmal or persistent sinus arrest with replacement by subsidiary escape rhythms in the atrium, AV junction, or ventricular myocardium.

Can manifest with:
- Sinus bradycardia
- Sinus arrhythmia—associated with SND in the elderly in the absence of respiratory pattern association.
- Sinoatrial exit block.
- Sinus arrest—pause >3 seconds.
- Atrial fibrillation with slow ventricular response.
- Bradycardia–tachycardia syndrome **(Fig. 6)**.

Chapter 7: Bradyarrhythmias

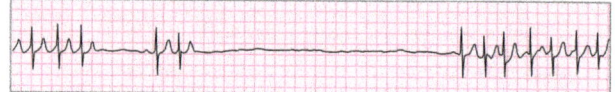

Fig. 6: Electrocardiogram showing sinus node dysfunction.

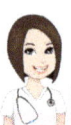

Nursing Considerations

- Monitor the vital signs.
- Place the patient on a cardiac monitor
- Obtain an ECG
- Assess the oxygenation status and serum electrolyte levels.
- Advice the patient for bed rest.
- Auscultate the cardiac murmurs.
- Monitor the patient for fluid retention
- Maintain the I/O charting
- Observe the weight of the patient.
- Withhold medications that can disrupt cardiac rhythm (usually beta-blockers and anti-arrhythmics) if ordered.
- Educate the patient if undergoing pacemaker insertion.
- After surgery, educate the patient to keep the arm still and avoid strenuous activities.
- Ask the patient to always carry a medical alert bracelet.

Electrolytes and ECG

CHAPTER 8

INTRODUCTION

- The electrocardiogram (ECG) is an extremely sensitive method of detecting types of electrolyte imbalance.
- The form of the normal ECG depends upon the normal ionic constitution of the cells and, particularly, of the extracellular fluid bathing the cardiac cells.
- Any significant alteration in the electrolyte content of this fluid, or the ratio between them, may directly or indirectly produce significant electrocardiographic changes.
- The electrolytes that may produce the ECG changes are calcium and potassium.
- Alterations in magnesium levels also produce ECG changes
- Hyponatremia or hypernatremia per se does not affect the ECG, but indirectly changes the potassium effect by inducing acid-base imbalance and altering the potassium-to-sodium ratio.
- The severity of electrolyte imbalances can also, on some occasions, be estimated on the basis of the ECG changes
- Early recognition of this sign may contribute to rapid correction of electrolyte imbalance, preventing potential serious complications.

POTASSIUM DISORDERS

ECG Features of Hyperkalemia
- **Rhythm:** Atrial and ventricular rhythms are regular
- **Rate:** Atrial and ventricular rates are within normal limits

- **P-wave:** Mild-low amplitude, moderate-wide flattened, severe-indiscernible (absent)
- **PR interval:** Normal or prolonged; unmeasurable, if P wave cannot be detected
- **QRS complex:** Widened because ventricular depolarization takes longer
- **QT interval:** Shortened
- **ST segment:** May be elevated in severe hyperkalemia **(Table 1)**
- **T wave:** Tall, peaked **(Figs. 1 to 5)**

Potassium levels	Expected ECG changes
Mild hyperkalemia (5.5–6.5 mmol/L)	Tall "peaked" T waves with narrow QT
Moderate hyperkalemia (6.5–8.0 mmol/L)	Peaked T waves, prolonged PR interval, decreased amplitude of P waves, widening of QRS complex
Severe hyperkalemia (>8.0 mmol/L)	Absence of P waves, intraventricular blocks, widening of QRS complex, eventual "sine-wave" pattern, VF, asystole

Table 1: Different potassium levels and changes in ECG.

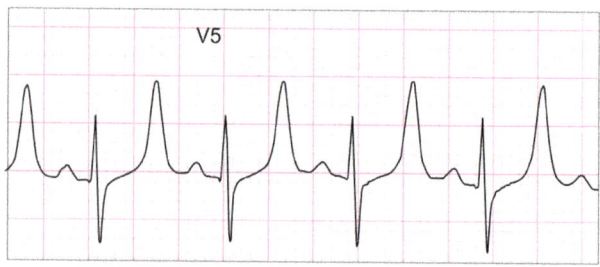

Fig. 1: Electrocardiogram showing peaked T waves in hyperkalemia.

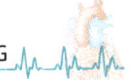

Chapter 8: Electrolytes and ECG

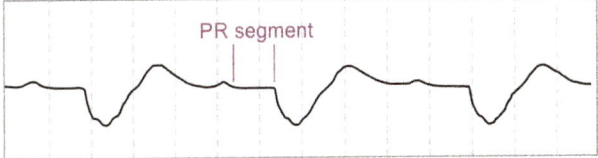

Fig. 2: Electrocardiogram showing prolonged PR segment and broad QRS in hyperkalemia.

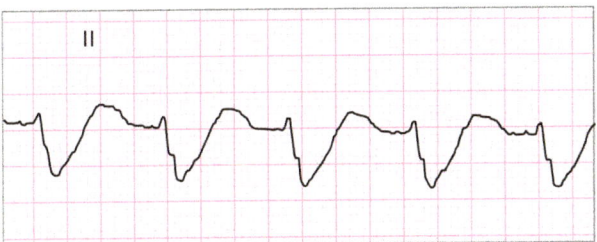

Fig. 3: Electrocardiogram showing loss of P waves and sine wave in severe hyperkalemia.

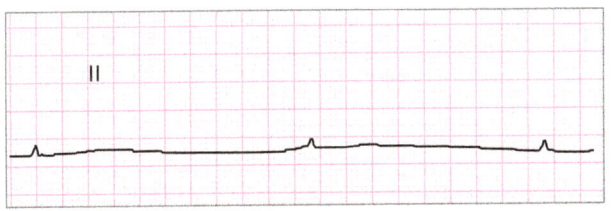

Fig. 4: Electrocardiogram showing severe bradycardia in hyperkalemia.

Chapter 8: Electrolytes and ECG

	ECG finding	Relative risk for adverse event (95% CI)
Normal		
Mild to moderate	Peaked T wave	0.77 (0.35–1.70)
	PR prolongation	4.11 (0.88–19.28)
Severe	QRS prolongation (bundle branch block, NSIVCD)	4.74 (2.01–11.15)
	2nd-degree heart block	6.92 (4.88–9.82)
Killer B's of HyperK: Broad Brady Blocks Bizarre	3rd-degree heart block	NA
	Junctional rhythm	7.46 (4.32–12.87)
	Ventricular escape rhythm	7.67 (5.28–11.13)
	Bradycardia (HR <50 bpm)	12.29 (6.69–22.57)
	Bizarre morphology, sine wave appearance, STEMI mimics	NA
	Ventricular tachycardia, ventricular fibrillation	NA

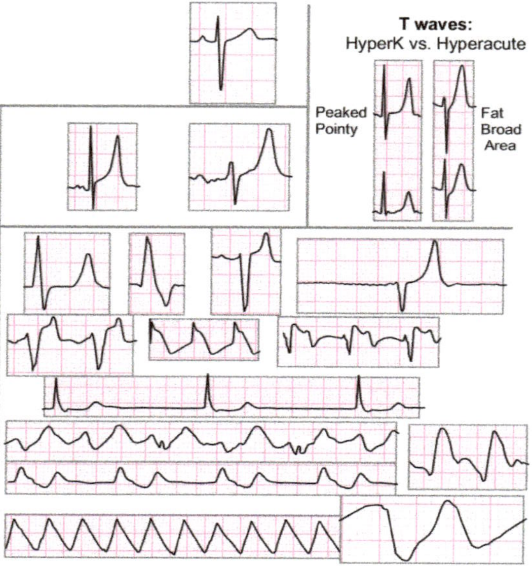

Fig. 5: Hyperkalemia ECG findings.

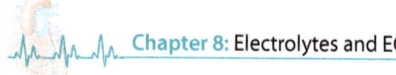

ECG Features of Hypokalemia

- **Rhythm:** Atrial and ventricular rhythms are regular
- **Rate:** Atrial and ventricular rates are within normal limits
- **P wave:** Prominent
- **PR interval:** May be prolonged
- **QRS complex:** Within normal limits or possibly widened; prolonged in hypokalemia
- **QT interval:** Usually indiscernible as T wave flattens
- **ST segment:** Depressed
- **T wave:** Amplitude is decreased. Inverted T wave
- **U wave may appear.** QU interval is prolonged **(Figs. 6 and 7)**

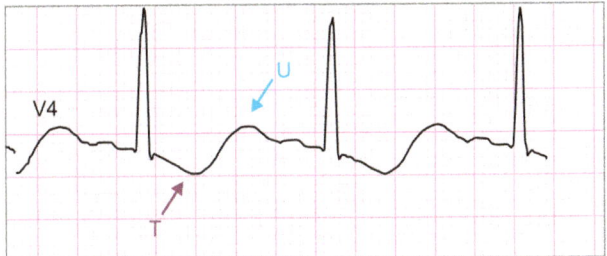

Fig. 6: Electrocardiogram showing T inversion and prominent U wave in hypokalemia.

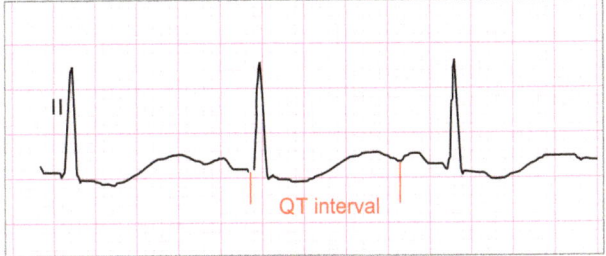

Fig. 7: Electrocardiogram showing long QT interval in hypokalemia.

Hypokalemia also predisposes to various tachyarrhythmias similar to antiarrhythmic drugs, such as quinidine and digitalis—most commonly ventricular ectopics.

CALCIUM DISORDERS

ECG Features of Hypocalcemia

- **Atrial and ventricular rhythm:** Regular
- **Atrial and ventricular rate:** Within normal limits
- **P-wave:** Normal
- **PR interval:** Normal
- **QRS complex:** Normal
- **QT interval:** Prolonged
- **ST segment:** Prolonged
- **T- wave:** Normal or flattened

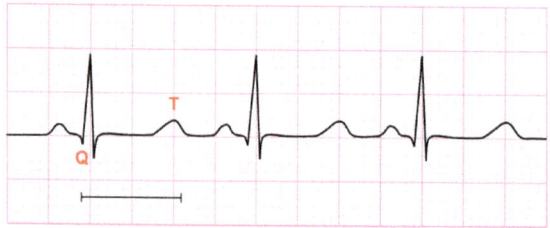

Fig. 8: ECG showing prolonged QT interval in hypocalcemia.

ECG Features of Hypercalcemia

- **Atrial and ventricular rhythm:** Regular
- **Atrial and ventricular rate:** Normal or bradycardia
- **P-wave:** Normal
- **PR interval:** Prolonged
- **QRS complex:** Normal or prolonged
- **QT interval:** Shortened
- **ST segment:** Normal
- **T-wave:** Normal

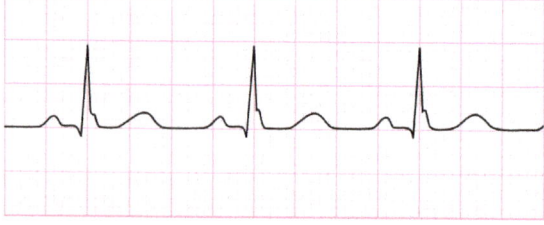

Fig. 9: ECG showing shortened QT interval in hypercalcemia.

Chapter 8: Electrolytes and ECG

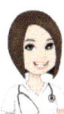

Nursing Considerations

- Monitor the pulse rate and BP
- Keep strict intake/output chart
- Blood samples for electrolytes, ABG, renal functions to be sent
- Make list of medications patient is on
- Counsel patient regarding need ICU care, continuous ECG monitoring and hemodialysis if needed

Drugs and Miscellaneous

DIGOXIN EFFECT

- Downsloping ST depression with a characteristic "reverse tick" or "Salvador Dali sagging" appearance (**Fig. 1**).

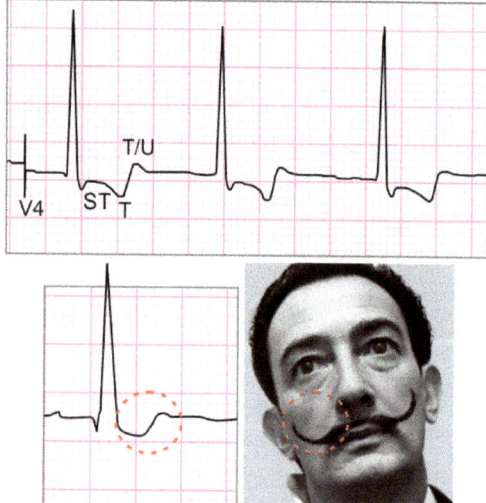

Fig. 1: Digoxin effect showing "reverse tick".

- Flattened, inverted, or biphasic T waves
- Shortened QT interval
- Mild PR interval prolongation
- Prominent U waves

MISCELLANEOUS

PERICARDITIS (FIGS. 2 TO 4)

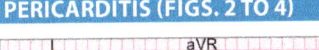

Fig. 2: ECG showing pericarditis.

- Widespread concave ST elevation and PR depression throughout most of the limb leads (I, II, III, aVL, aVF) and precordial leads (V2-6)
- Reciprocal ST depression and PR elevation in lead aVR (± V1)

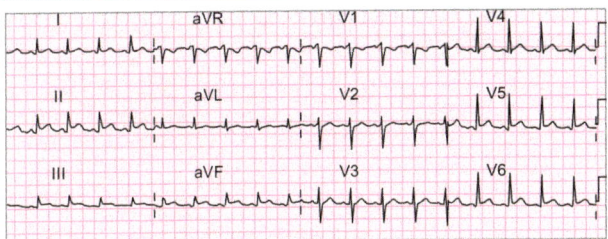

Figs. 3A and B: Reciprocal ST depression and PR elevation in pericarditis.

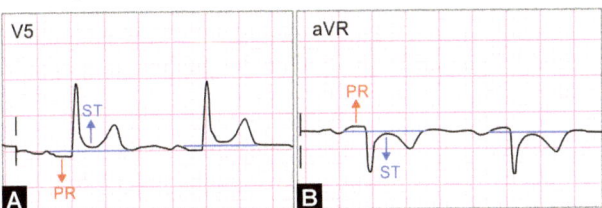

Fig. 4: ECG changes in acute pericarditis.

PULMONARY EMBOLISM

- Sinus tachycardia: The most common abnormality (44%)
- Complete or incomplete right bundle branch block (RBBB) (18%)

Chapter 9: Drugs and Miscellaneous

- Right ventricular strain pattern: T inversions in the right precordial leads and the inferior leads
- Dominant R wave in V1: A manifestation of acute right ventricular dilatation (16%)
- P pulmonale (9%)

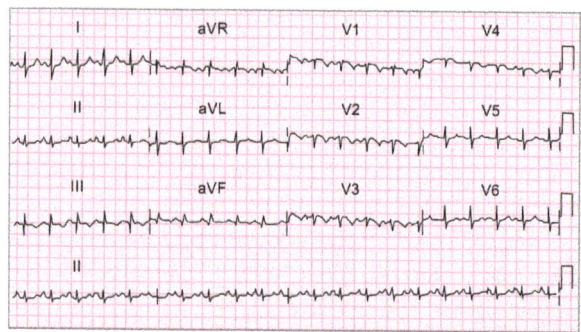

- **SI QIII TIII pattern:** Deep S wave in lead I, Q wave in III, inverted T wave in III (20%). This "classic" finding is neither sensitive nor specific for PE—**McGinn and White sign (Figs. 5A and B).**

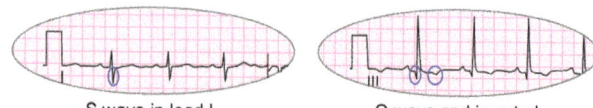

S wave in lead I   Q wave and inverted T wave in lead III

Figs. 5A and B: McGinn and White sign.

List of drugs causing QT prolongation.

- Antiarrhythmics (e.g., amiodarone)
- Antibiotics (e.g., erythromycin, clarithromycin)
- Antidepressants (e.g., citalopram, escitalopram)
- Antifungals (e.g., fluconazole, voriconazole)
- Antihistamines (e.g., cetirizine, fexofenadine)
- Antipsychotics (e.g., haloperidol, risperidone)
- Methadone
- Ondansetron
- Domperidone
- Hydroxyzine

PACING IN ECG

The term "pacing" in ECG refers to the electrical stimulation of the heart muscle by a pacemaker device. A pacemaker is a small device that is implanted under the skin in the chest or abdomen with wires that are threaded through a vein into the heart. The pacemaker sends electrical impulses to the heart muscle to regulate the heartbeat when the heart's natural pacemaker (the sinoatrial node) is not working properly. The pacing rate can be adjusted by a physician to ensure that the heart is beating at a steady and appropriate rate.

Atrial Pacing

ECG of atrial pacing shows a pacing spike followed by a P wave that is different from the sinus P wave. This is because the pacemaker is artificially initiating the heartbeat from the atria instead of the natural sinoatrial (SA) node. The QRS complex and T wave may also be altered depending on the underlying heart disease and the type of pacemaker used.

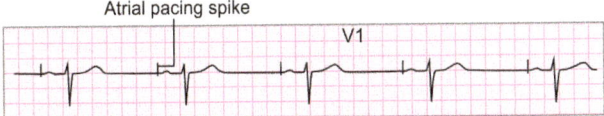

Atrial pacing with normal conduction to the ventricles via atrioventricular system. The ventricles are depolarized via the bundle of His-Purkinje network, resulting in the normal QRS complex duration.

Ventricular Pacing

An ECG of ventricular pacing shows a pacing spike followed by a QRS complex that is different from the normal QRS complex. This is because the pacemaker is artificially initiating the heartbeat from the ventricles instead of the natural SA node. The P wave may be absent or dissociated from the QRS complex.

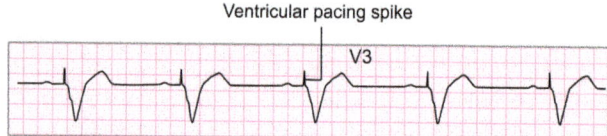

Ventricular pacing spike — V3

Spontaneous atrial activity is sensed by the atrial lead and triggers ventricular stimulations. The QRS complex is wide due to ventricular depolarization proceeding outside the conduction system.

Atrial and Ventricular Pacing

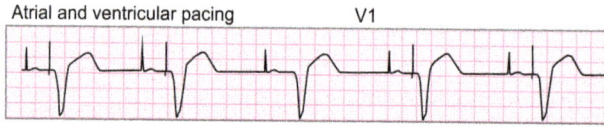

Atrial and ventricular pacing — V1

Pacing in the right atrium and the right ventricles.

Review—Multiple Choice Questions

CHAPTER 10

1. **The P-wave of normal ECG:**
    A. Has voltage and duration nearly equal 2.5 × 2.5 mm.
    B. Is upright in aVR.
    C. Represents right atrial depolarization in its second half.
    D. Inverted in lead II.

2. **In regard to Q wave all the followings are correct, *except*:**
    A. Represents septal depolarization from left to right in V5.
    B. Its depth is not more than 1/4 its corresponding R.
    C. Its duration is not more than 0.04 seconds.
    D. Deep and wide Q is seen in recent myocardial infarction.

3. **In normal ECG:**
    A. The average duration of QT interval is 0.50 seconds.
    B. The ST segment is an isoelectric line.
    C. The T wave is rounded and symmetrical.
    D. The height of the T wave is >10 mm chest leads.

4. **Regarding the PR interval of the ECG, all the followings are correct, *except*:**
    A. Represents atrial depolarization and conduction through AV node.
    B. Normal duration from 0.12 to 0.20 second
    C. Prolonged in right bundle branch block
    D. Prolonged in 1st degree heart block.

Chapter 10: Review—Multiple Choice Questions

5. **Regarding the ECG findings in heart block (HB), all the followings are correct, *except*:**
   A. Complete (HB): Complete dissociation between P waves and QRS complexes.
   B. 1st degree (HB): PR interval is abnormally long.
   C. 2nd degree (HB): A ventricular beat may follow every 2nd or 3rd atrial beat.
   D. 1st degree (HB): PR interval lengthens progressively until a ventricular beat is dropped.

6. **True statement regarding the ECG of ventricular hypertrophy (VH):**
   A. Axis of the heart is from −30 to +90 degrees in right VH.
   B. S wave in V1 or V2 plus R wave in V5 or V6 account > 35 mm in left VH in adults.
   C. S wave is deep in V1 and V2 and R wave is tall in V5 and V6 in right VH.
   D. Right VH may occur in systemic hypertension.

7. **A delay in the AV node is indicated by a P-R interval:**
   A. Between 0.12 and 0.20 seconds
   B. Between 0.04 and 0.12 seconds
   C. Less than 0.12 seconds
   D. Greater than 0.20 seconds

8. **Which of the following is not a characteristic feature of normal sinus rhythm?**
   A. Irregular rhythm
   B. P-R interval of 0.16 seconds
   C. QRS duration of 0.08 seconds
   D. Rate of 60–100
   E. P wave before the QRS complex

9. **Lead V5 is placed at:**
   A. Left anterior axillary line in 5th intercoastal space (ICS).
   B. Left midclavicular line in 4th ICS.
   C. Left midclavicular line in 5th ICS.
   D. Left midaxillary line in 5th ICS.

10. The rate of discharge in case of bundle of His pacemaker is:
   A. 40–60/min
   B. 20–30/min
   C. 60–80/min
   D. 30–40/min

11. With normal standardization, each 1 mm represents:
   A. 0.1 mV
   A. 0.01 mV
   B. 1 mV
   C. 10 mv

12. What is the normal range of the QRS axis?
   A. 0 to 180 degrees
   B. 0 to +90 degrees
   C. −30 to +110 degrees
   D. −90 to +90 degrees
   E. −90 to +30 degrees

13. Determine the QRS axis for the ECG shown in Figure 1:

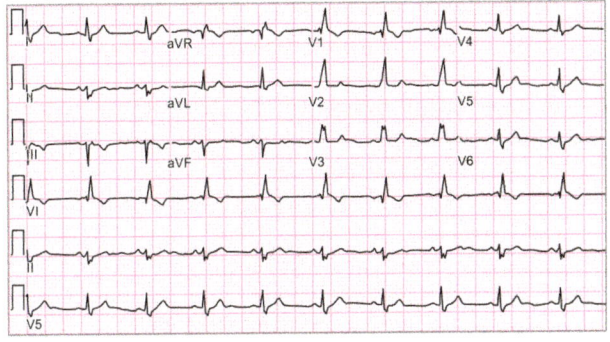

Fig. 1: ECG 1.

   A. −60 degrees
   B. +45 degrees
   C. +60 degrees
   D. Indeterminate
   E. 0 degree

14. Determine the QRS axis for the ECG shown in Figure 2:

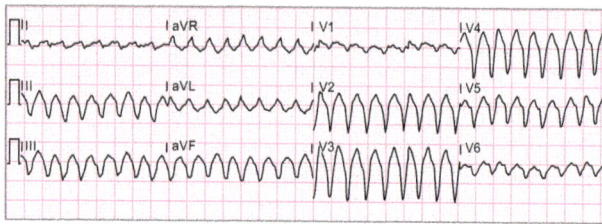

Fig. 2: ECG 2.

A. Normal axis
B. Right axis deviation
C. Left axis deviation
D. Extreme axis deviation

15. The combination of right axis deviation and left ventricular diastolic overload with atrial fibrillation is suggestive of:
A. Mitral stenosis
B. Mitral incompetence
C. Aortic stenosis
D. Pulmonary incompetence

16. The cause of right axis deviation are all, *except*:
A. Left pneumothorax
B. Anterolateral myocardial infarction (MI)
C. Inferior MI
D. Left posterior fascicular block

17. The most common cause for left axis deviation is:
A. Left anterior hemiblock
B. left bundle branch block (LBBB)
C. Left ventricular hypertrophy
D. Q waves of inferior myocardial infarction

18. Which of the following statements about the ECG are true?
A. The P wave of the ECG reflects atrial contraction
B. The P-Q interval is normally about 0.1 second.
C. The QRS complex reflects the ventricular depolarization.

Chapter 10: Review—Multiple Choice Questions

D. The T-wave reflects the repolarization of the Purkinje fibers

19. Regarding the causes of the ECG waves all the following are correct, *except*:
   A. P-wave by atrial depolarization.
   B. QRS complex by ventricular depolarization.
   C. T wave by ventricular repolarization.
   D. U wave by papillary muscle depolarization.

20. The causes of the ECG "intervals". Which is false?
   A. PR by AV nodal conduction.
   B. ST by atrial repolarization.
   C. QT by ventricular depolarization and ventricular repolarization.

21. Axis of the heart all are true, *except*:
   A. Mean instantaneous vector of QRS complexes in vertical plane.
   B. Normally from −30 to +60.
   C. Deviated to left side in full-term pregnant woman.
   D. Deviated to right side in long-slender person

22. Left axis deviation of the ECG is described when:
   A. The axis of the heart is from −30 to +90 degree.
   B. The QRS complex is prominent positive in lead aVF.
   C. The QRS is prominent positive in lead I and prominent negative in lead III.
   D. Right ventricle is enlarged

23. What electrical event of the heart is NOT recorded on the standard 12-lead ECG trace?
   A. Atrial depolarization
   B. Atrial repolarization
   C. Ventricular depolarization
   D. Ventricular repolarization

24. The time necessary for ventricular depolarization is represented by the:
   A. P-R interval
   B. QRS interval

C. QT interval
D. S-T segment
E. QRS complex

25. **Which of the following ECG lead combinations can be used to evaluate the anterior and lateral walls of the left ventricle?**

    A. aVR and V1
    B. II, III, and aVF
    C. V3 and V4
    D. V5 and V6
    E. V3, V4, V5, and V6

26. **Identify the correct statement/s:**

    A. A segment is a straight line connecting two waves.
    B. An interval encompasses at least one wave plus the connecting straight line.
    C. An interval is a straight line connecting two waves.
    D. A segment encompasses at least one wave plus the connecting straight line.

27. **Ruling out limb lead reversal.**

    A. avR is always negative
    B. Lead I is always positive
    C. Lead II and III positive for the P wave and usually the QRS complex
    D. All of the above

28. **ECG description: Rate = ~150 bpm, irregularly irregular, baseline irregularity, no visible p waves, QRS occur irregularly with its length usually <0.12s. Diagnosis?**

    A. Atrial flutter
    B. Atrial fibrillation
    C. Ventricular tachycardia
    D. Supraventricular tachycardia

Chapter 10: Review—Multiple Choice Questions

29. Young male with episodic palpitations. ECG is given below. What is your diagnosis?

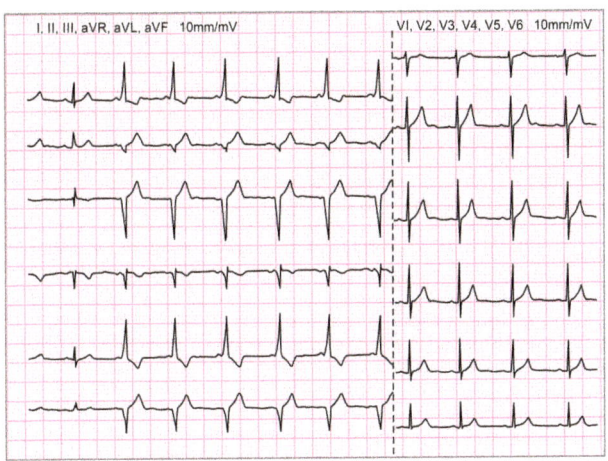

- A. Mobitz type 2 heart block
- B. Pre-excitation syndrome
- C. Acute pericarditis
- D. Hypocalcemia

30. Diagnosis.

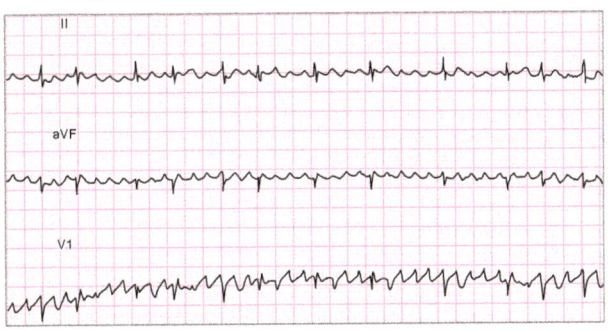

- A. Supraventricular tachycardia
- B. Atrial fibrillation
- C. Ventricular fibrillation
- D. Atrial flutter with variable blocks

31. A 60-year-old man complains that since 1 hour, he has been experiencing palpitations, a feeling of unease, and vague chest pain. The peripheral pulse is difficult to count because of the uneven amplitude and time span between beats; apical rate is 130 per minute, with only one heart sound evidence in many of the beats, blood pressure (BP) is 115–130/60–75, imprecise because the Korotkoff sound are inconsistent (his usual BP is 145/85). An ECG shows an electrical rate of 150, with clearly identifiable narrow QRS complexes, but an irregular baseline and no identifiable P waves. What will be the diagnosis?
    A. Ventricular tachycardia
    B. Atrial fibrillation
    C. Atrial flutter
    D. Supraventricular tachycardia

32. Diagnosis.

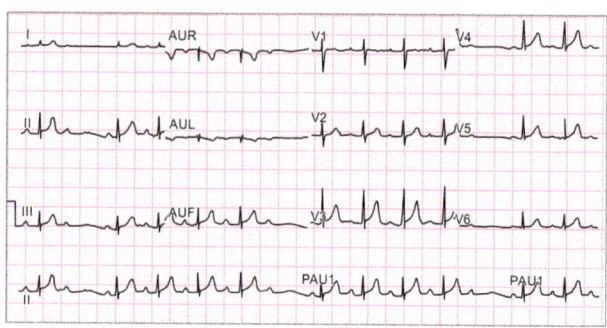

    A. First degree heart block
    B. Second degree heart block—Mobitz type 1
    C. Second degree heart block—Mobitz type 2
    D. Third degree heart block

33. All the followings cause low voltage ECG, *except*:
    A. Hypothermia
    B. Body mass index (BMI) >35

C. Hypothyroidism
D. Hypokalemia

34. Match causes of sudden cardiac death with their ECG findings.

1. RSR' with STE in V1-3	a. WPW
2. RVH, Epsilon waves	b. Brugada syndrome
3. Delta wave, short PR	c. Hypertrophic obstructive cardiomyopathy (HOCM)
4. Voltage criteria for left ventricular hypertrophy (LVH), precordial T wave inversion, "dagger" Q waves.	d. Arrhythmogenic right ventricular dysplasia

A. 1b, 2d, 3a, 4c
B. 1c, 2d, 3a, 4b
C. 1b, 2c, 3d, 4a
D. 1a, 2b, 3c, 4d

35. The ECG findings in electrolyte imbalance:

A. Tall and peaked T wave in hypokalemia.
B. T wave inversion and prominent U wave in hyperkalemia.
C. Prolonged QT interval in hypocalcemia.
D. ST elevation in hyponatremia.

36. What is/are the etiology of the wide QRS?

A. Sinus rhythm with complete left bundle branch block
B. Accelerated idioventricular rhythm
C. A-V sequential pacing
D. Atrial sensed and ventricular paced pattern
E. All of the above

37. Which one of the following is associated with ST segment elevation in ECG?

A. Left ventricular hypertrophy (LVH)
B. Right ventricular hypertrophy (RVH)
C. Digoxin effect
D. Early repolarization after an attack of angina
E. Subendocardial infarction

Chapter 10: Review—Multiple Choice Questions

38. Diagnosis.

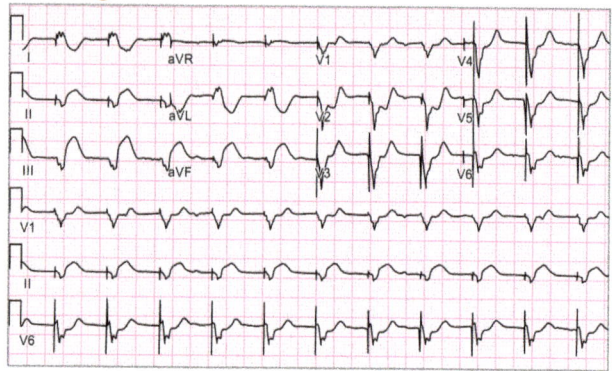

A. Inferior wall myocardial infarction (IWMI) with pacing
B. Anterior wall myocardial infarction (AWMI)
C. Benign early repolarization
D. Pericarditis

39. Diagnosis.

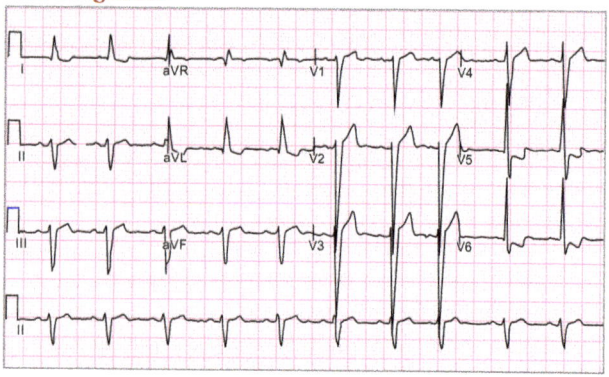

A. Right ventricular hypertrophy (RVH)
B. Left ventricular hypertrophy (LVH)
C. Hyperkalemia
D. Pericarditis

40. Diagnosis.

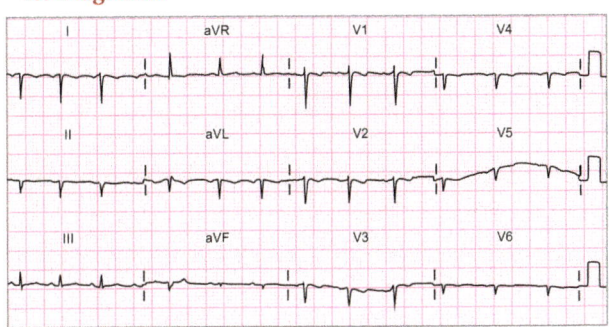

- A. Limb lead reversal
- B. Dextrocardia
- C. Normal ECG
- D. Atrial fibrillation

41. Elderly lady comatose.

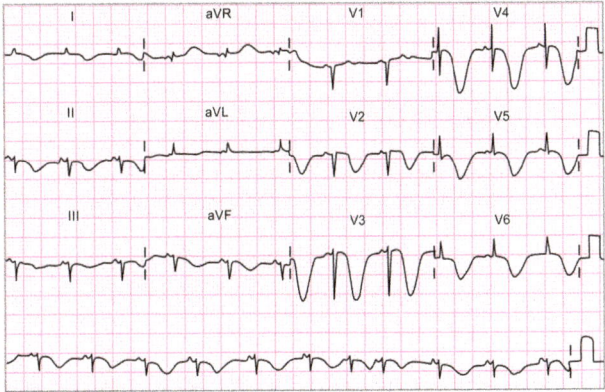

- A. Acute MI
- B. Hypoglycemia
- C. SAH
- D. Hypothermia

Chapter 10: Review—Multiple Choice Questions

42. Which is the drug of choice for the patient with the given ECG?

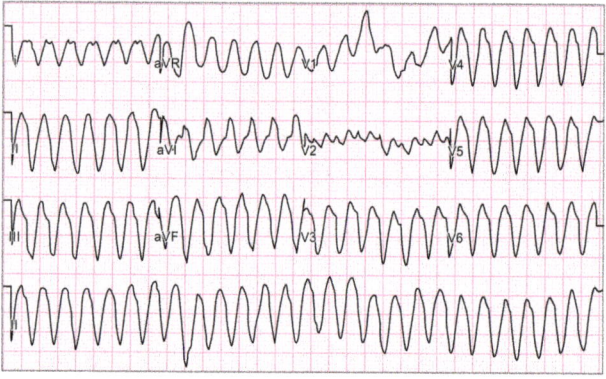

A. Verapamil
B. Sotalol
C. Lignocaine
D. Digitalis

43. Match the following.

1. First degree heart block	a. Saw-tooth pattern on baseline
2. Atrial fibrillation	b. Prolonged P-R interval
3. Atrial flutter	c. Some P waves are not followed by a QRS complex
4. Second-degree heart block	d. No P waves but an irregular baseline

A. 1b, 2d, 3a, 4c
B. 1c, 2d, 3a, 4b
C. 1b, 2c, 3d, 4a
D. 1a, 2b, 3c, 4d

Chapter 10: Review—Multiple Choice Questions

44. A 25-year-old male presented with crush injury after road traffic accident (RTA).

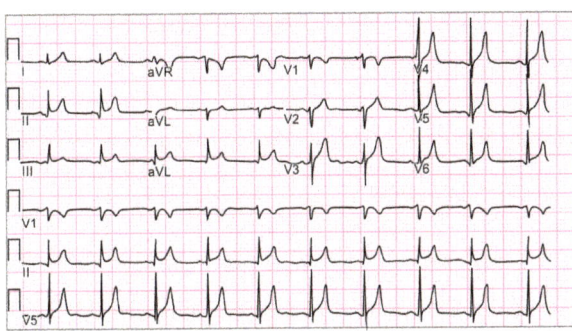

A. Acute ST elevation MI
B. Acute pericarditis with tamponade
C. Acute kidney injury with hyperkalemia
D. Acute respiratory distress syndrome

45. The ECG shown below is consistent with which of the following clinical situations?

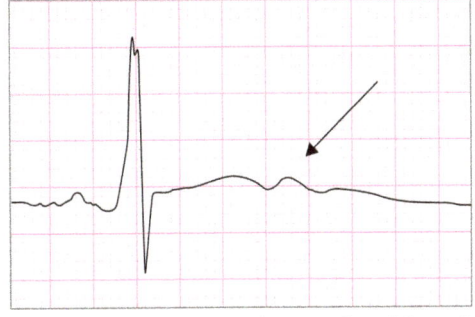

A. A 55-year-old man complaining of crushing substernal chest pain
B. A 25-year-old woman with acute renal failure resulting from plus nephritis
C. A 27-year-old man with prolonged neutropenia after induction therapy for acute myelogenous leukemia (AML) who is receiving amphotericin B.
D. A 57-year-old woman with metastatic breast cancer receiving etidronate.

46. Diagnosis.

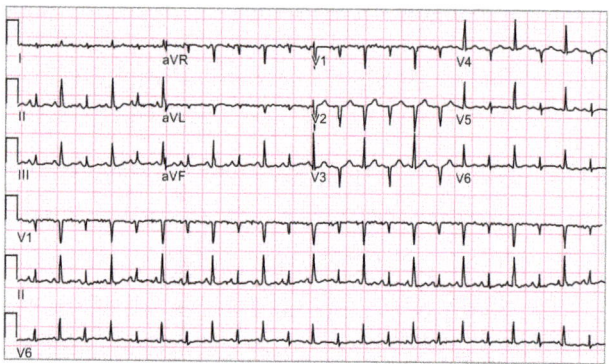

- A. Sinus tachycardia
- B. Atrial fibrillation
- C. Electrical alternans
- D. Supraventricular tachycardia

47. A 13-year-boy presented with central cyanosis, clubbing, and multiple heart sounds.

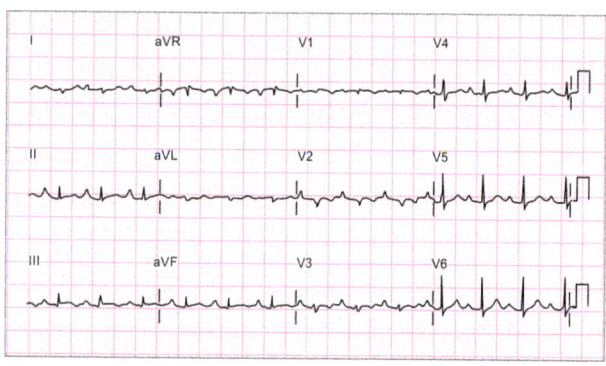

- A. Atrial septal defect (ASD)
- B. Ventricular septal defect (VSD)
- C. Tetralogy of Fallot (TOF)
- D. Ebstein

Chapter 10: Review—Multiple Choice Questions

48. Findings of the ECG:

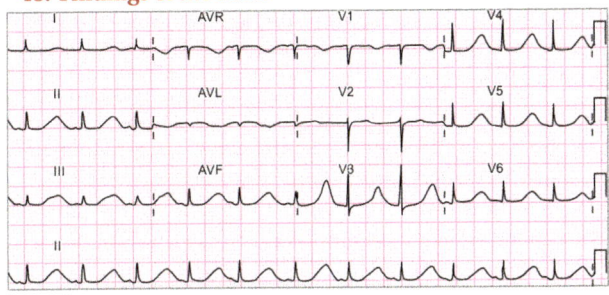

A. Short PR, prolonged QRS, normal QT
B. Normal PR, normal QRS, normal QT
C. Normal PR, normal QRS, long QT
D. Prolonged PR, normal QRS, normal QT

49. A 75-year-old smoker presenting with dyspnea and productive cough.

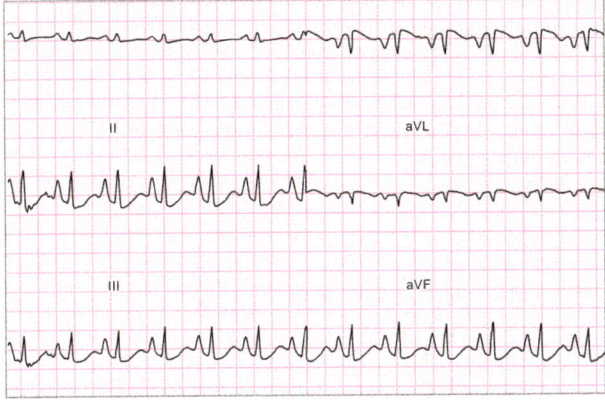

A. Atrial fibrillation
B. Sinus tachycardia, right atrial enlargement (RAE)
C. Supraventricular tachycardia, left atrial enlargement (LAE)
D. Normal ECG

Chapter 10: Review—Multiple Choice Questions

50. All of the following conditions are more commonly associated with left bundle branch block (LBBB) pattern than right bundle branch block (RBBB) pattern on ECG, *except:*
    A. Acute MI
    B. Aortic valve disease
    C. Lev disease
    D. ASD

51. Idiopathic degeneration of the proximal bundle branch fibers is known as:
    A. Lev's disease
    B. Lenegre's disease
    C. Ashman phenomenon
    D. Brugada syndrome

52. All of the following may occur due to hyperkalemia, *except*:
    A. Prolonged PR interval
    B. Prolonged QRS interval
    C. Prolonged QT interval
    D. Ventricular asystole

53. Pseudo-P-Pulmonale is typically seen in:
    A. Hypokalemia
    B. Hyponatremia
    C. Hypocalcemia
    D. Hypercalcemia

54. QT prolongation is seen in all, *except*:
    A. Hypothermia
    B. Digitalis toxicity
    C. Hypocalcemia
    D. Romano–Ward syndrome

55. Which of the following is not associated with prolonged QT interval syndrome?
    A. Romano–Ward syndrome
    B. Jervell and Lange Nielsen syndrome
    C. Flecainide therapy
    D. Lidocaine therapy

Chapter 10: Review—Multiple Choice Questions

56. Prolonged QT interval is seen in all of the following, *except*:
   A. Hypokalemia
   B. Hypocalcemia
   C. Use of macrolide antibiotics
   D. Hypernatremia

57. Hypocalcemia is characterized by all of the following features, *except*:
   A. Numbness and tingling of circumoral region
   B. Hyperactivity tendon reflexes
   C. Shortening of Q-T interval in ECG
   D. Carpopedal spasm

58. All of the following electrocardiographic findings may represent manifestations of digitalis intoxication, *except*:
   A. Bigeminy
   B. Junctional tachycardia
   C. Atrial flutter
   D. Parasystole

59. Osborne waves in ECG are seen in:
   A. Hypothyroidism
   B. Hypothermia
   C. Hypocalcemia
   D. Hypokalemia

60. Nobel Prize for invention of ECG was awarded to:
   A. Hewlet
   B. Judkin
   C. Einthoven
   D. White

61. A mean QRS axis of −30 to −60 degree is seen in:
   A. Left ventricle hypertrophy
   B. Right ventricle hypertrophy
   C. Left posterior fascicular block
   D. Lateral wall myocardial infarction

62. The normal P wave is inverted in lead:
   A. Lead I
   B. Lead II

C. aVF
D. aVR

63. Absent P wave is seen in:

A. Atrial fibrillation
B. Cor pulmonale
C. Mitral stenosis
D. COPD

64. Which of the following is the order of activation after stimulation of Purkinje fibers is?

a. Septum > Endocardium > Epicardium
b. Endocardium > Septum > Epicardium
c. Epicardium > Septum > Endocardium
d. Septum > Epicardium > Endocardium

65. A QRS duration between 100 and 120 milliseconds suggests all of the following, *except*:

A. First degree AV block
B. Left anterior fascicular block
C. Left posterior fascicular block
D. Left bundle branch block

66. Wide QRS complex may be seen in all of the following, *except*:

A. Hyperkalemia
B. Wolf-Parkinson-White syndrome
C. Ventricular tachycardia
D. Mobitz type 2 AV block

67. Wide QRS complex is typically seen in:

A. Bundle branch block
B. Sick sinus syndrome
C. Mobitz type I block
D. Mobitz type II block

68. Low QRS voltage on ECG with left ventricular hypertrophy on echocardiography suggests a diagnosis of:

A. Pericardial effusion
B. Cardiac amyloidosis
C. Cor pulmonale
D. Infective endocarditis

Chapter 10: Review—Multiple Choice Questions

69. In left ventricular hypertrophy (LVH), SVI + RV5 is more than_how much.........mV?
    A. 2.5mV
    B. 3.0 mV
    C. 3.5 mV
    D. 4.0 mV

70. ST elevation is seen in all of the following conditions, *except*:
    A. Myocardial infarction
    B. Coronary artery spasm
    C. Ventricular hypertrophy
    D. Ventricular aneurysm
    E. Early repolarization variant
    F. Prinzmetal angina

71. What is the diagnostic of fresh myocardial infarction in ECG?
    A. QT interval prolongation
    B. P mitrale
    C. ST segment elevation
    D. ST segment depression

72. Reciprocal changes in ECG in patients with inferior wall myocardial infarction are seen in which leads?
    A. Lead aVL
    B. Lead II
    C. Lead III
    D. Lead aVF

73. The following ECG changes are associated with hypokalemia:
    A. Severe ST segment depression
    B. Increased amplitude and width of the P wave
    C. Prolongation of the PR interval
    D. Increased height ratio of the U wave compared to the T wave
    E. All of the above

74. These conditions can cause the tall T waves seen in ECG, *except*:
    A. Hyperkalemia
    B. Ischemia

C. Early repolarization
D. Normal variant

75. The following ECG changes are associated with hyperkalemia:
A. Pseudo right bundle branch block with ST elevation
B. P wave becomes more prominent in the anterior lead
C. Ventricular tachycardia
D. Sinus tachycardia

76. ECG changes in hyperkalemia are associated with:
A. Slower repolarization that will create tall T waves with a narrow base
B. Inactivation of sodium channels
C. Hyperactivity of potassium channels
D. Faster conduction of electrical activity

ANSWERS

1. A	2. D	3. B	4. C	5. D
6. B	7. D	8. A	9. A	10. D
11. A	12. C	13. A	14. D	15. B
16. C	17. A	18. A, C	19. D	20. B
21. B	22. C	23. B	24. E	25. E
26. A, B	27. D	28. B	29. B	30. D
31. B	32. B	33. D	34. A	35. C
36. E	37. E	38. A	39. B	40. B
41. C	42. C	43. A	44. C	45. C
46. C	47. D	48. C	49. B	50. D
51. A	52. C	53. A	54. B	55. D
56. D	57. C	58. D	59. B	60. C
61. A	62. D	63. A	64. A	65. A
66. D	67. A	68. B	69. C	70. C
71. C	72. A	73. E	74. D	75. C
76. A				

Practice ECGs

CASE SCENARIO-1

A 50-year-old diabetic patient presented with history of acute onset of dyspnea since 3 hours.

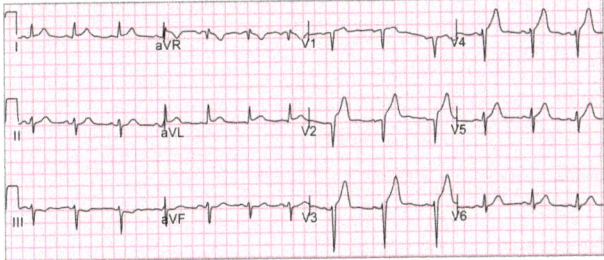

Rate	71
Rhythm	Regular
Axis	Left
P wave	Normal
PR interval/segment	Normal
QRS	Narrow, QS complexes in septal leads
ST segment	Elevation in I, aVL, v2, depression in III ('South African flag' sign), elevations seen in v1–4
T wave	Hyperacute T waves seen in v2–3
QT interval	0.348
Final diagnosis	Hyperacute anteroseptal MI

CASE SCENARIO-2

A 24-year-old male with 2 days of central chest pain now complains of dyspnea.

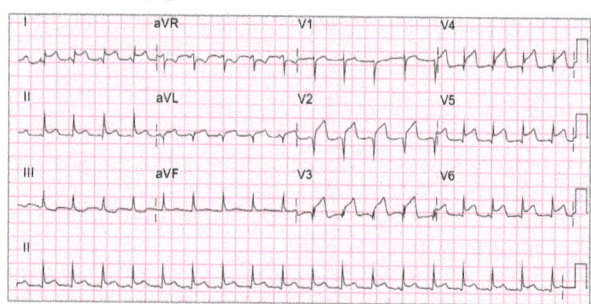

12-lead ECG showing

Rate	110 bpm
Rhythm	Sinus rhythm
Axis	Normal
P wave	Duration 0.08 sec and normal morphology
PR interval/ segment	• 0.12 sec • PR segment elevation in aVR
QRS	0.08 sec
ST segment	• Elevation in V2–6, I, aVL • Depression in aVR
T wave	Normal
QT interval	0.32 sec
Final diagnosis	Acute pericarditis

Chapter 11: Practice ECGs

CASE SCENARIO-3

A 60-year-old male chronic smoker presents with sudden onset giddiness and hypotension.

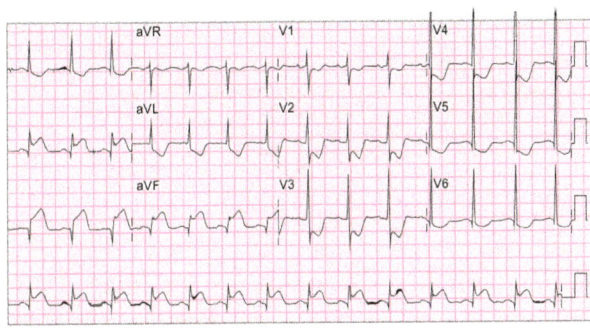

12-lead ECG showing

Rate	85 bpm
Rhythm	Sinus
Axis	Normal
P wave	Duration 0.12 sec and normal morphology
PR interval/segment	0.16 sec
QRS	0.08 sec, dominant R wave in v1–3
ST segment	• Elevation in II, III, and aVF (elevation in lead III > II) • Depression in V1–6, I, aVL
T wave	Corresponds to ST–T changes
QT interval	0.36 sec
Final diagnosis	Inferior wall myocardial infarction (MI) with extension to posterior wall

Chapter 11: Practice ECGs

CASE SCENARIO-4

A 26-year-old female with episodic palpitations.

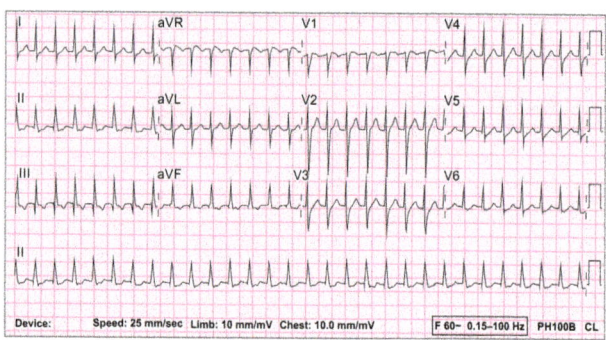

12-lead ECG showing

Rate	200 bpm
Rhythm	Regular
Axis	Normal
P wave	Retrograde
PR interval/ segment	–
QRS	0.08 sec (narrow complex)
ST segment	Normal
T wave	Normal
QT interval	0.28 sec
Final diagnosis	Supraventricular tachycardia-atrioventricular nodal reentry tachycardia (SVT-AVNRT)

CASE SCENARIO-5

A 65-year-old male with history of ischemic heart disease (IHD), now complains of syncope.

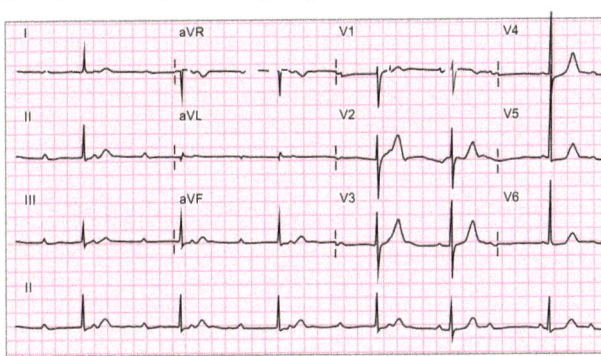

12-lead ECG showing

Rate	Atrial—80 bpm; ventricular—50 bpm
Rhythm	Junctional escape
Axis	Normal
P wave	Present
PR interval/segment	–
QRS	0.08 sec independent of P waves
ST segment	Normal
T wave	Normal
QT interval	0.36 sec
Final diagnosis	Complete heart block

CASE SCENARIO-6

A 34-year-old female with history of irregular palpitations on exertion.

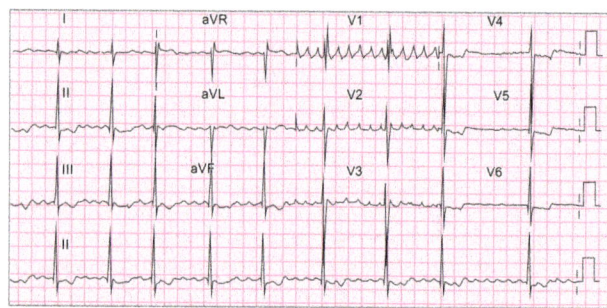

12-lead ECG showing

Rate	70 bpm (6-second rule)
Rhythm	Irregular
Axis	Normal
P wave	Absent, presence of fibrillatory waves
PR interval/ segment	–
QRS	0.08 sec varying RR interval
ST segment	Normal
T wave	Normal
QT interval	0.32 sec
Final diagnosis	Atrial fibrillation (coarse AF)

CASE SCENARIO-7

A 45-year-old male brought to the casualty in an unresponsive state.

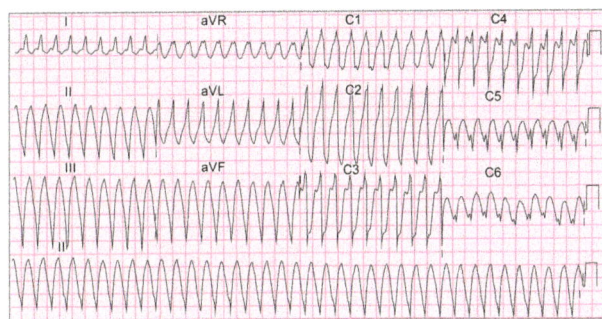

12-lead ECG showing

Rate	250 bpm
Rhythm	Regular
Axis	Left-northwest
P wave	AV dissociation
PR interval/ segment	–
QRS	0.28 sec (broad complex); positive concordance
ST segment	–
T wave	–
QT interval	–
Final diagnosis	Monomorphic ventricular tachycardia (VT)

CASE SCENARIO-8

A 60-year-old male, smoker complains of palpitations and lightheadedness.

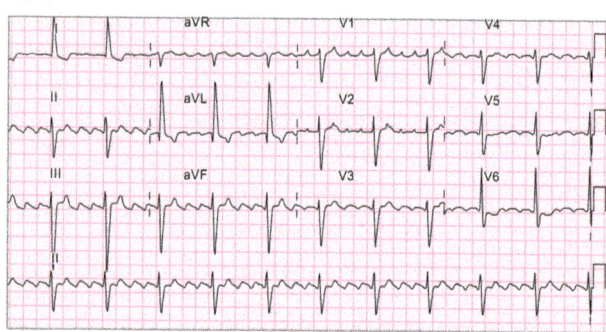

Rate	Atrial ~250; ventricular ~65
Rhythm	Regular
Axis	Leftward
P wave	"Saw-tooth" pattern
PR interval/segment	No PR interval
QRS	Narrow
ST segment	Cannot be commented
T wave	Superimposed by flutter waves
QT interval	Cannot be commented
Final diagnosis	• **Atrial flutter** with fixed AV block (4:1) • LVH (limb lead voltage criteria: R in aVL ≥13 mm, S in III ≥15 mm, R in I+S in III >25 mm)

CASE SCENARIO-9

A 34-year-old lady with RHD presents for regular follow-up.

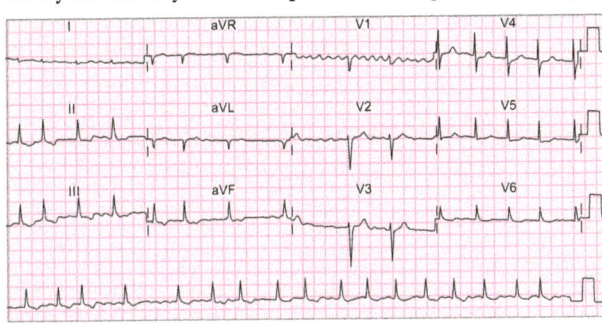

Rate	102 (number of complexes in 10 sec rhythm strip x 6)
Rhythm	Irregular
Axis	Normal
P wave	Absent, coarse fibrillary waves (V1)
PR interval/ segment	Cannot be commented
QRS	Narrow
ST segment	ST segment depression with downward slopping in II, III, aVF
T wave	Normal
QTc interval	0.443
Final diagnosis	• **Atrial fibrillation** with rapid ventricular response • Digoxin effect ("sagging" ST depressions in inferior leads)/ MI (reciprocal ST depressions of a high-lateral MI) (Note: If on digoxin for atrial fibrillation, then the rate here is uncontrolled)

Chapter 11: Practice ECGs

CASE SCENARIO-10

A 70-year-old female presented with fatigue.

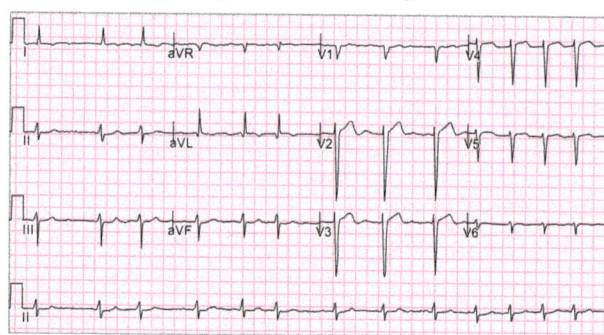

Rate	78 (number of complexes in 10 sec rhythm strip x 6)
Rhythm	Irregular
Axis	Leftward
P wave	Absent, fine fibrillary waves (v1)
PR interval/segment	Cannot be commented
QRS	Narrow, poor R wave progression
ST segment	Normal
T wave	Flat/inverted in lateral leads
QTc interval	0.410
Final diagnosis	• **Atrial fibrillation** • Possible old lateral wall MI

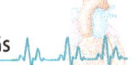

Chapter 11: Practice ECGs

CASE SCENARIO-11

A 24-year-old asymptomatic male underwent ECG for pre-employment screening.

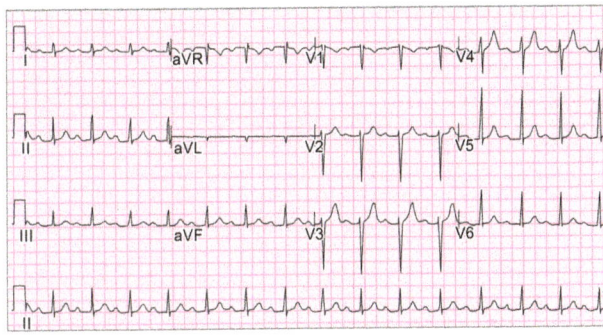

Rate	88
Rhythm	Regular
Axis	Normal
P wave	Normal
PR interval/segment	0.28, prolonged
QRS	Narrow
ST segment	Normal
T wave	Normal
QTc interval	0.436
Final diagnosis	1st degree AV block

CASE SCENARIO-12

A 42-year-old hypertensive man presented with episode of pre-syncope.

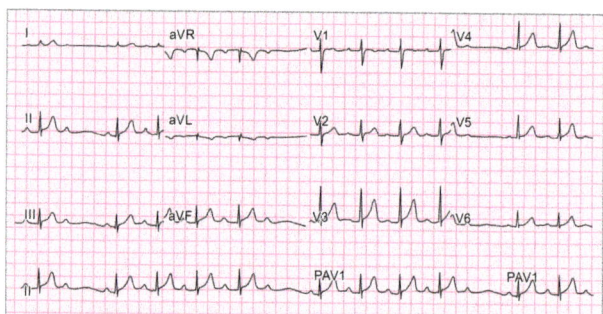

Rate	88
Rhythm	Regular sinus with dropped beat at regular intervals
Axis	Normal
P wave	Normal
PR interval/segment	Progressive prolongation of PR interval with subsequent non-conducted P wave
QRS	Narrow
ST segment	Normal
T wave	Normal
QTc interval	0.388
Final diagnosis	2nd degree AV block Mobitz type 1 (Wenckebach phenomenon)

CASE SCENARIO-13

A 70-year-old male was found unconscious in the jogging park.

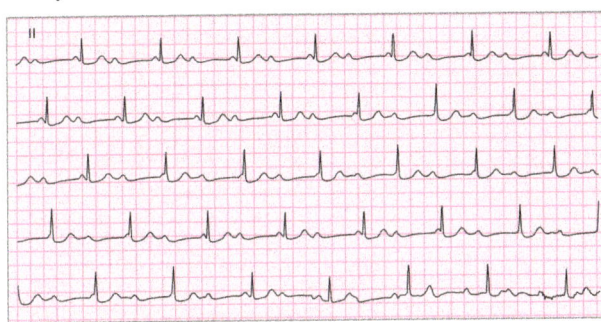

Rate	Atrial—88; ventricular—42
Rhythm	Regular, junctional escape
Axis	Single lead cannot comment
P wave	Normal
PR interval/ segment	Varying, isorhythmic AV dissociation (some P waves appear to conduct, but on closer inspection the PR interval is varying. What appears to be a relationship between the P waves and QRS complexes is purely by chance)
QRS	Narrow
ST segment	Depressions with upsloping (nonspecific)
T wave	Normal
QTc interval	0.418
Final diagnosis	3rd degree (complete) heart block

CASE SCENARIO-14

A 34-year-old male gets ECG done for pre-employment purpose.

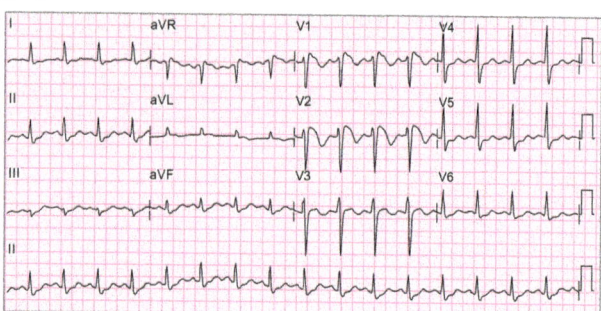

Rate	100
Rhythm	Regular
Axis	Normal
P wave	Normal
PR interval/segment	Normal
QRS	Narrow, rSR' in v1, v2
ST segment	Coved ST elevation in v1, v2 ST depressions in other leads
T wave	T wave inversions in v1, v2, and v3
QTc interval	0.516
Final diagnosis	• **Brugada syndrome (type 1)** • Hypokalemia to be considered (generalized ST depressions, QT prolongation, type 1 Brugada-like pattern)

CASE SCENARIO-15

A 55-year-old male with chronic obstructive pulmonary disease (COPD) admitted to the ICU with worsening dyspnea.

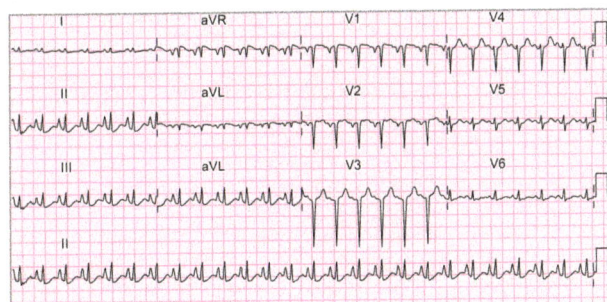

Rate	150
Rhythm	Regular
Axis	Normal
P wave	Tall (>2.5; P pulmonale)
PR interval/segment	Normal
QRS	Narrow, poor R wave progression, lead 1 sign of emphysema
ST segment	Normal
T wave	Normal
QTc interval	0.443
Final diagnosis	**Right atrial enlargement** (possible etiology being cor-pulmonale)

Chapter 11: Practice ECGs

CASE SCENARIO-16

A 20-year-old male athlete gets ECG done before traveling abroad.

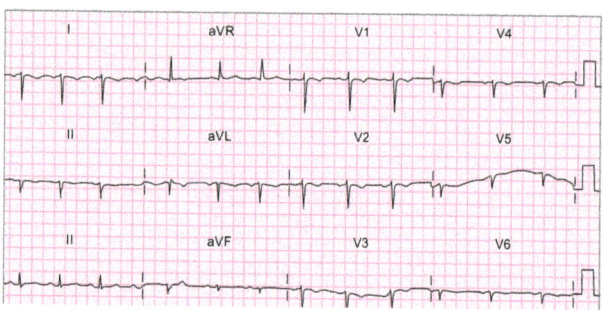

Rate	75
Rhythm	Regular
Axis	Northwest
P wave	Normal, inverted in most leads
PR interval/segment	Normal
QRS	Narrow, upright in lead aVR, poor R wave progression
ST segment	Normal
T wave	Inverted in most leads
QTc interval	0.358
Final diagnosis	Dextrocardia

CASE SCENARIO-17

A 24-year-old male with road traffic accident (RTA) and crush injury admitted to the ICU.

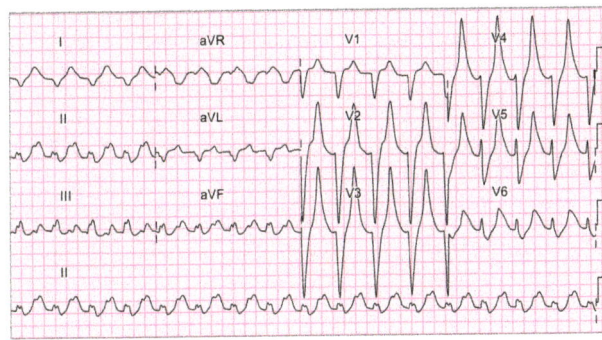

Rate	~100
Rhythm	Regular
Axis	Right
P wave	Flattened (barely seen)
PR interval/ segment	Cannot be commented
QRS	Broad bizarre looking merged
ST segment	Elevations/depressions seen (appropriate discordance)
T wave	Tall peaked (tented)
QT interval	Difficult to comment (almost sine wave-like pattern seen)
Final diagnosis	Severe hyperkalemia

CASE SCENARIO-18

A 37-year-old male presented with fatigue and quadriparesis. He had similar episodes two times in the past.

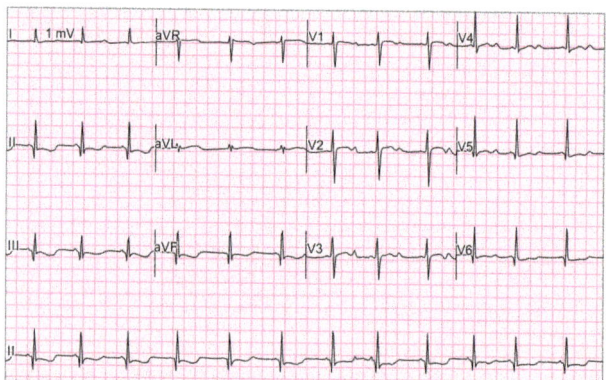

Rate	68
Rhythm	Regular
Axis	Normal
P wave	Normal
PR interval/ segment	Normal
QRS	Narrow, prominent Q waves in inferior leads
ST segment	Depressions in inferior leads
T wave	Flattening
QTc interval	0.511, prominent U waves seen (apparent QT prolongation)
Final diagnosis	• **Severe hypokalemia** • Possible old inferior wall MI

CASE SCENARIO-19

A 65-year-old male undergoes yearly health checkup.

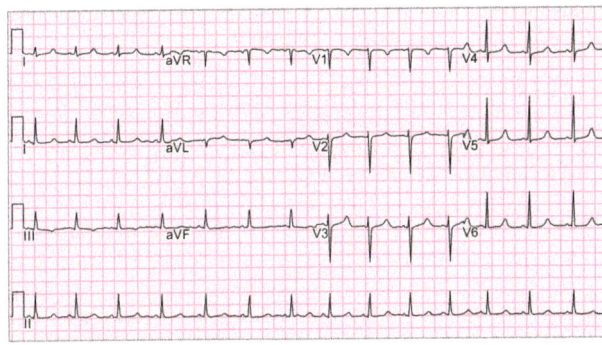

Rate	83
Rhythm	Regular
Axis	Normal
P wave	Normal
PR interval/segment	Normal
QRS	Narrow
ST segment	Normal
T wave	Normal
QTc interval	0.470
Final diagnosis	Normal ECG

CASE SCENARIO-20

A 68-year-old hypertensive male presented with altered sensorium. His CT scan revealed large hemorrhage in internal capsule with intraventricular extension.

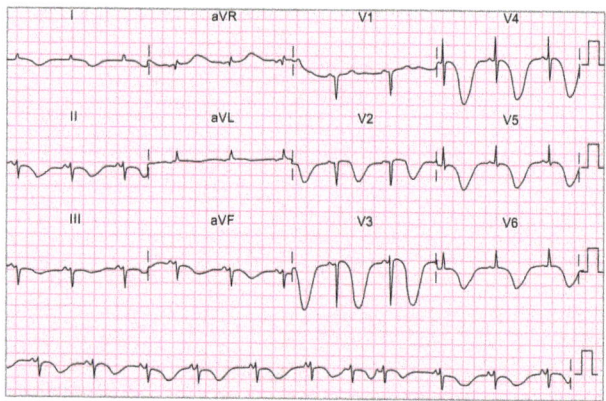

Rate	63
Rhythm	Regular
Axis	Left
P wave	Normal
PR interval/segment	Normal
QRS	Narrow
ST segment	Normal
T wave	Widespread deep inversions (cerebral T waves)
QTc interval	0.600
Final diagnosis	Features favor raised intracranial tension

CASE SCENARIO-21

A 60-year-old female presented with severe left-sided chest pain since 4 hours.

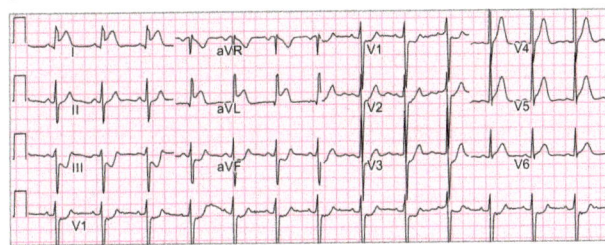

Rate	88
Rhythm	Regular
Axis	Left
P wave	Normal
PR interval/segment	Normal
QRS	Narrow
ST segment	Elevations in I, aVL; reciprocal depressions in II, III, and aVF; depressions in v1–3 (reciprocal changes or anterior ischemia)
T wave	Normal
QTc interval	0.388
Final diagnosis	Acute **high-lateral wall STEMI** with possible anteroseptal ischemia

CASE SCENARIO-22

A 40-year-old male posted for hernia surgery underwent ECG for preoperative evaluation.

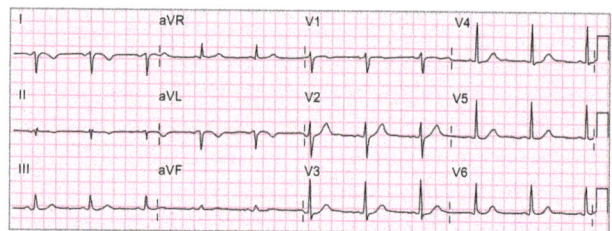

Rate	60
Rhythm	Regular
Axis	Right
P wave	Normal
PR interval/segment	Normal
QRS	Narrow, normal R wave progression, and upright in lead aVR
ST segment	Normal
T wave	Normal
QTc interval	0.41
Final diagnosis	Incorrect lead (limb lead) placement

Chapter 11: Practice ECGs

CASE SCENARIO-23

A 47-year-old male presented with chest discomfort.

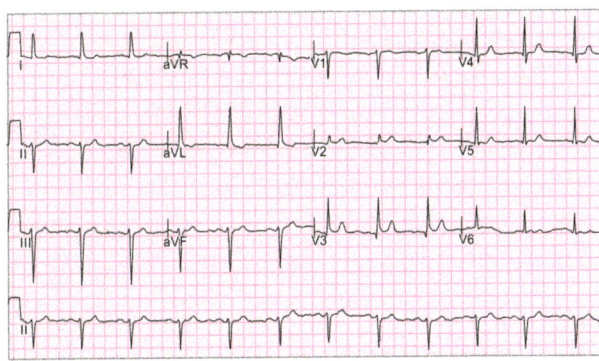

Rate	75
Rhythm	Regular
Axis	Left
P wave	Normal
PR interval/ segment	Normal
QRS	Narrow, q waves in v2–3
ST segment	Subtle elevations in anteroseptal leads
T wave	Normal
QTc interval	0.402
Final diagnosis	• LVH (limb lead voltage criteria: R in aVL ≥13 mm, S in III ≥15 mm, R in I+S in III >25 mm) • Possible anteroseptal MI (although changes are not very specific, it should be suspected in the presence of any q waves anterior/septal leads)

CASE SCENARIO-24

A 50-year-old female found unresponsive at home.

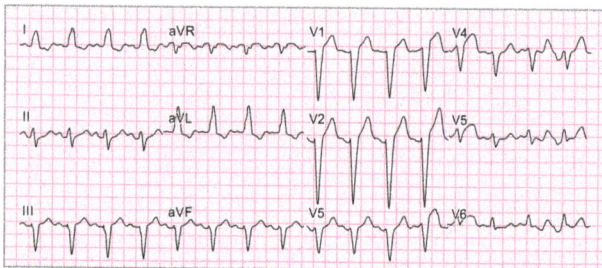

Rate	100
Rhythm	Regular
Axis	Left
P wave	Normal
PR interval/segment	Normal
QRS	Wide (140 ms), deep S in v1, tall slurred R best seen in I, aVL, absent q in v5-6
ST segment	Elevations/depressions seen (appropriate discordance)
T wave	Normal
QT interval	0.465
Final diagnosis	LBBB, rule out ACS

CASE SCENARIO-25

A 48-year-old male found hypertensive on regular follow up.

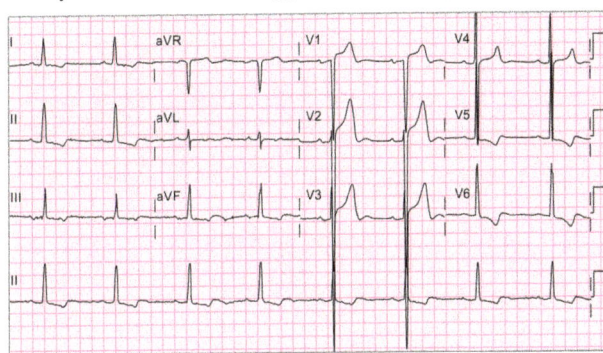

Rate	50
Rhythm	Regular
Axis	Normal
P wave	Normal
PR interval/ segment	Normal
QRS	Narrow
ST segment	Down sloping depressions in all leads with dominant R wave
T wave	Inversions seen all leads with dominant R wave (strain pattern)
QT interval	0.402
Final diagnosis	Left ventricular hypertrophy with LV strain sinus bradycardia

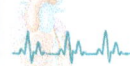

Chapter 11: Practice ECGs

CASE SCENARIO-26

A 50-year-old farmer presented with chronic cough and dyspnea on exertion.

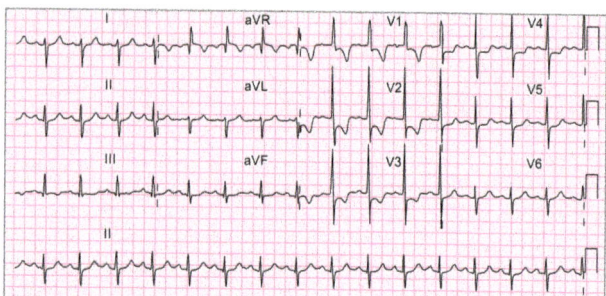

Rate	94
Rhythm	Regular
Axis	Right
P wave	Normal
PR interval/segment	Normal
QRS	Narrow, tall R in v1 (>7 mm, R/S ratio >1), deep S in v6 (>7 mm, R/S ratio <1)
ST segment	Depressions in v1–4
T wave	Inversions in v1–4
QT interval	0.451
Final diagnosis	Right ventricular hypertrophy with RV strain pattern

CASE SCENARIO-27

A 50-year-old female admitted for evaluation of anasarca and fatigue.

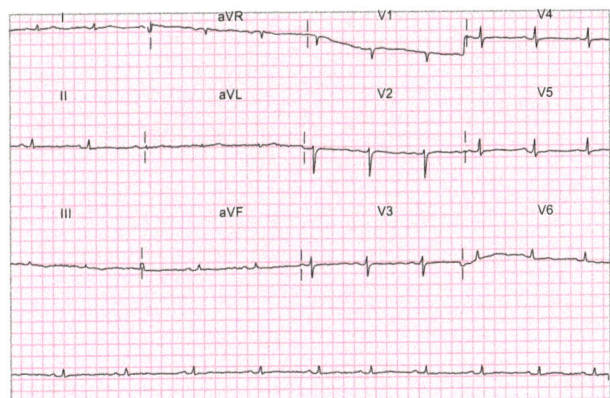

Rate	68
Rhythm	Regular
Axis	Normal
P wave	Normal
PR interval/ segment	Normal
QRS	Narrow, low-voltage complexes in all limb leads (<5 mm)
ST segment	Normal
T wave	Generalized flattening
QTc interval	0.383 (T waves are barely visible. T waves in leads I and III used for calculation)
Final diagnosis	**Low QRS voltage** with possible etiology being hypothyroidism

CASE SCENARIO-28

A 55-year-old male presented with a recent history of inferior wall MI comes for follow up after 1 month.

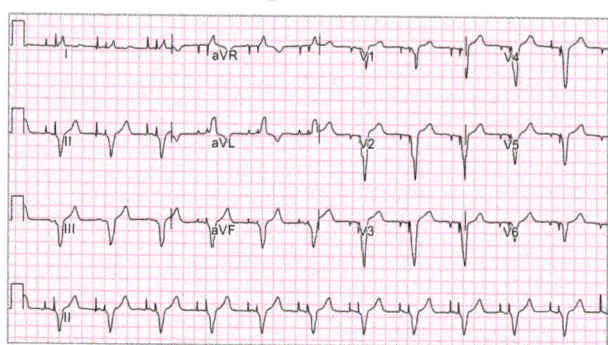

Rate	71
Rhythm	Regular, pacemaker spikes seen—atrial and ventricular with complete capture.
Axis	Left
P wave	Small, normal morphology succeeding each atrial pacemaker spike
PR interval/ segment	Normal
QRS	Broad with nonspecific interventricular conduction block morphology (but may be taken as LBBB morphology, note deep slurred S in v1)
ST segment	Normal
T wave	Normal
QT interval	0.479
Final diagnosis	A-V sequential pacing (ventricular pacemaker lead more likely in RV)

Chapter 11: Practice ECGs

CASE SCENARIO-29

A 26-year-old male is seen in out-patient department (OPD). His brother had sickle cell disease (SCD) 2 weeks ago.

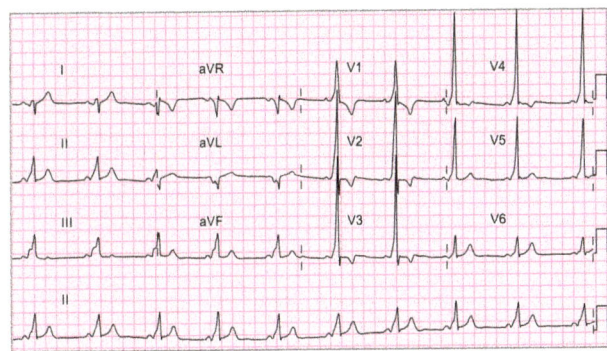

Rate	60
Rhythm	Regular
Axis	Normal/rightward
P wave	Normal
PR interval/ segment	Short (<120 ms)
QRS	Wide (~ 160 ms), slurring of upstroke ('Delta' wave), dominant R wave in v1, apparent Q wave in lead aVL (this is actually a negative delta wave, which simulates a lateral wall MI, hence the name "pseudo-infarction" pattern)
ST segment	Normal
T wave	Inverted in v1-3 (tall R with t wave inversions in septal leads mimics RVH, but these changes are due to repolarization abnormalities and not RVH)
QTc interval	0.440
Final diagnosis	Wolff–Parkinson–White (WPW) syndrome (type A)

CASE SCENARIO-30

A 46-year-old female post-lower (uterine) segment cesarean section (LSCS) complains of acute dyspnea.

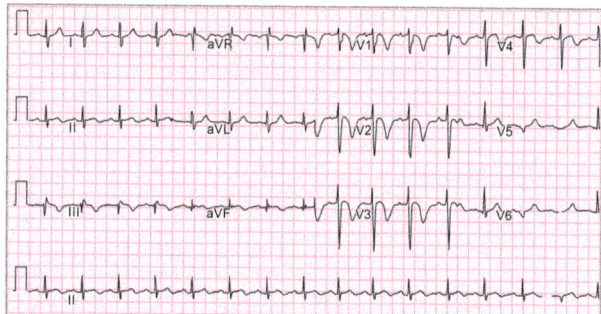

Rate	94
Rhythm	Regular
Axis	Normal
P wave	Normal
PR interval/segment	Normal
QRS	Narrow
ST segment	Nonspecific changes in lead III
T wave	Inversions in v1–3, II, III, and aVF (RV strain pattern)
QT interval	0.350
Final diagnosis	Features favor pulmonary embolism (note also the S1Q3T3 pattern)

CASE SCENARIO-31

A 39-year-old female admitted for cholecystectomy. Her preoperative ECG is done.

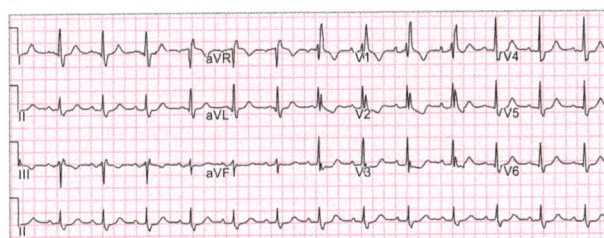

Rate	79
Rhythm	Regular
Axis	Normal
P wave	Normal
PR interval/ segment	Normal
QRS	Wide, rSR' in v1–2, deep wide slurred S in v5–6 and I
ST segment	Normal
T wave	Inversions in v1–2 (appropriate discordance)
QTc interval	0.413
Final diagnosis	Right bundle branch block (RBBB)

CASE SCENARIO-32

A 20-year-old marathon runner got an ECG done for medical checkup.

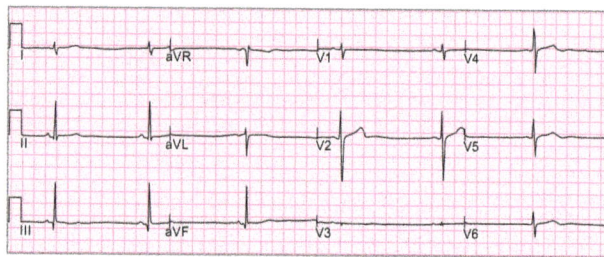

Rate	~37
Rhythm	Regular
Axis	Normal
P wave	Normal
PR interval/segment	Normal
QRS	Narrow
ST segment	Normal
T wave	Normal
QTc interval	0.346
Final diagnosis	Sinus bradycardia

Chapter 11: Practice ECGs

INTERPRET ECG

ECG 1

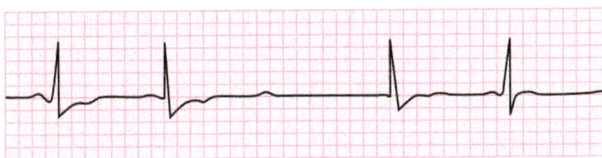

Atrial rhythm
Ventricular rhythm
Atrial rate
Ventricular rate
P-wave
PR interval
QRS complex
T-wave
QT interval
Interpretation

ECG 2

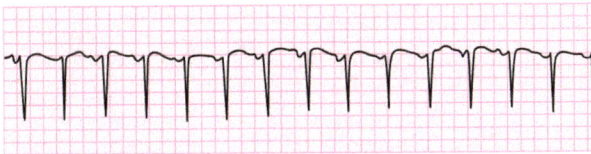

Atrial rhythm
Ventricular rhythm
Atrial rate
Ventricular rate
P-wave
PR interval
QRS complex
T-wave
QT interval
Interpretation

Chapter 11: Practice ECGs

ECG 3

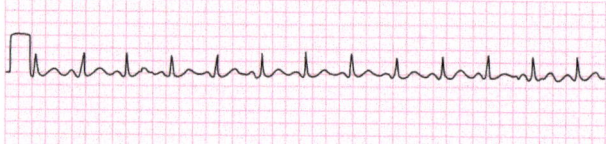

Atrial rhythm
Ventricular rhythm
Atrial rate
Ventricular rate
P-wave
PR interval
QRS complex
T-wave
QT interval
Interpretation

ECG 4

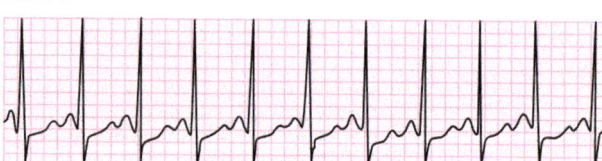

Atrial rhythm
Ventricular rhythm
Atrial rate
Ventricular rate
P-wave
PR interval
QRS complex
T-wave
QT interval
Interpretation

ECG 5

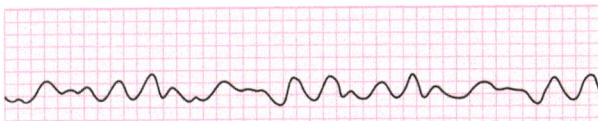

Atrial rhythm
Ventricular rhythm
Atrial rate
Ventricular rate
P-wave
PR interval
QRS complex
T-wave
QT interval
Interpretation

ANSWERS

ECG 1

Atrial rhythm	:	Regular
Ventricular rhythm	:	Irregular
Atrial rate	:	50 bpm
Ventricular rate	:	40 bpm
P-wave	:	Normal
PR interval	:	0.16 sec
QRS complex	:	0.08 sec
T wave	:	Normal
QT interval	:	0.40 sec
Interpretation	:	Type-II second degree AV block

ECG 2

Atrial rhythm	:	Regular
Ventricular rhythm	:	Regular
Atrial rate	:	150 bpm
Ventricular rate	:	150 bpm
P-wave	:	Peaked

PR interval	:	0.12 sec
QRS complex	:	0.08 sec
T wave	:	Flattened
QT interval	:	0.24 sec
Interpretation	:	Atrial tachycardia

ECG 3

Atrial rhythm	:	Regular
Ventricular rhythm	:	Regular
Atrial rate	:	125 bpm
Ventricular rate	:	125 bpm
P-wave	:	Normal
PR interval	:	0.14 sec
QRS complex	:	0.08 sec
T wave	:	Normal
QT interval	:	0.32 sec
Interpretation	:	Sinus tachycardia

ECG 4

Atrial rhythm	:	Regular
Ventricular rhythm	:	Regular
Atrial rate	:	110 bpm
Ventricular rate	:	110 bpm
P-wave	:	Normal
PR interval	:	0.16 sec
QRS complex	:	0.10 sec
T wave	:	Normal
QT interval	:	0.36 sec
Interpretation	:	Sinus tachycardia

ECG 5

Atrial rhythm	:	Cannot be determined.
Ventricular rhythm	:	Cannot be determined.
Atrial rate	:	Unmeasurable
Ventricular rate	:	Unmeasurable
P-wave	:	Absent
PR interval	:	Absent
QRS complex	:	Unmeasurable
T wave	:	Opposite to QRS complex
QT interval	:	Absent
Interpretation	:	Ventricular fibrillation

Chapter 11: Practice ECGs

FIND THE DIFFERENCE

(A)

Strip 1

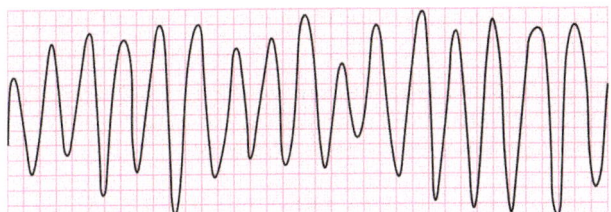

Strip 2

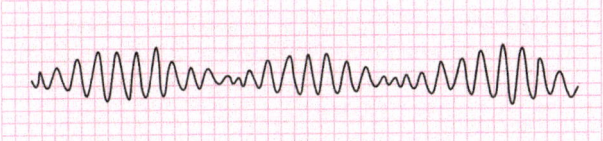

(B)

Strip 1

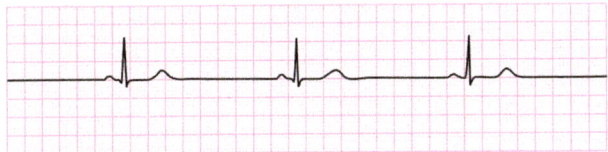

Strip 2

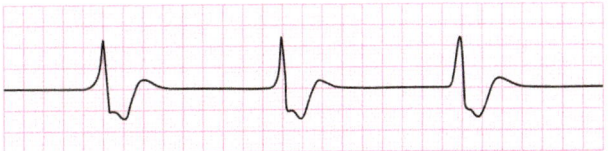

Answers

(A)

Strip 1: Ventricular flutter, smooth sine-wave appearance, it is a rapid, regular, repetitive beating of the ventricles. It is produced by a single ventricular focus firing at a rapid rate of 250 to 350 beats/minute.

Strip 2: Torsades de pointes, spindle-shaped appearance, it is variant form of ventricular tachycardia, with a rapid ventricular rate ranges between 250–350 beats/minute.

(B)

Strip 1: Sinus bradycardia, condition in which the sinus node creates an impulse at a slower-than-normal rate.

Strip 2: Idioventricular rhythm, also called ventricular escape rhythm, occurs when the impulse starts in the conduction system below the AV node. In the ECG, QRS complex appears bizarre.

Appendices

APPENDIX 1

Adult Tachycardia with a Pulse Algorithm

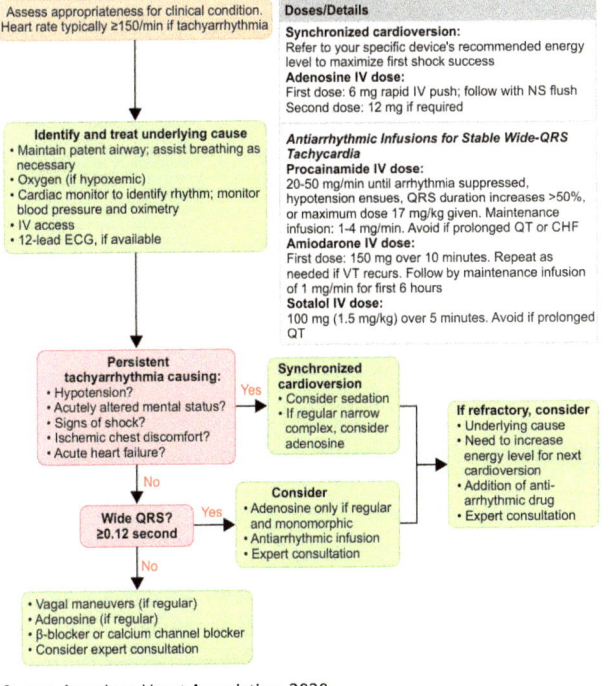

Source: American Heart Association, 2020.

Appendices

APPENDIX 2

Adult Bradycardia Algorithm

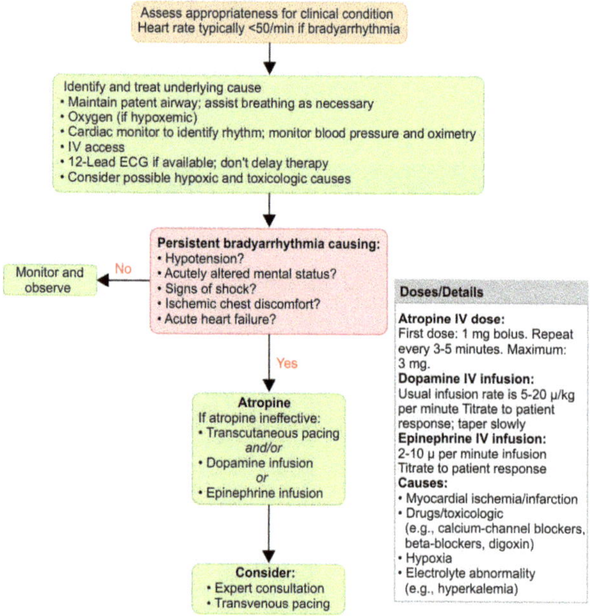

```
Assess appropriateness for clinical condition
Heart rate typically <50/min if bradyarrhythmia
                    ↓
Identify and treat underlying cause
• Maintain patent airway; assist breathing as necessary
• Oxygen (if hypoxemic)
• Cardiac monitor to identify rhythm; monitor blood pressure and oximetry
• IV access
• 12-Lead ECG if available; don't delay therapy
• Consider possible hypoxic and toxicologic causes
                    ↓
Persistent bradyarrhythmia causing:
• Hypotension?
• Acutely altered mental status?
• Signs of shock?
• Ischemic chest discomfort?
• Acute heart failure?
     No → Monitor and observe
     Yes ↓
Atropine
If atropine ineffective:
• Transcutaneous pacing
  and/or
• Dopamine infusion
  or
• Epinephrine infusion
                    ↓
Consider:
• Expert consultation
• Transvenous pacing
```

Doses/Details

Atropine IV dose:
First dose: 1 mg bolus. Repeat every 3-5 minutes. Maximum: 3 mg.
Dopamine IV infusion:
Usual infusion rate is 5-20 μg/kg per minute Titrate to patient response; taper slowly
Epinephrine IV infusion:
2-10 μ per minute infusion Titrate to patient response
Causes:
• Myocardial ischemia/infarction
• Drugs/toxicologic (e.g., calcium-channel blockers, beta-blockers, digoxin)
• Hypoxia
• Electrolyte abnormality (e.g., hyperkalemia)

Source: American Heart Association, 2020.

APPENDIX 3

Intrinsic Rates of Conduction System

Part of conduction system	Rate
Sinoatrial node	60–100 times/min
Atrioventricular node	40–60 times/min
Bundle of His, Purkinje fibers	20–40 times/min

APPENDIX 4

Condition	ECG changes
Hypokalemia	Prominent U-waves
Hyperkalemia	Peaked T-wave
Tricyclic antidepressant poisoning	Wide QRS complex
Acute myocardial infarction	ST segment elevation
Coronary ischemia	Flattened or inverted T-waves
Hypercalcemia	Shortened QT interval
Hypocalcemia	Prolonged QT interval

APPENDIX 5

Normal ECG Values of Waves and Intervals

RR interval	0.6–1.2 seconds
P-wave	80 milliseconds
PR interval	120–200 milliseconds
PR segment	50–120 milliseconds
QRS complex	80–100 milliseconds
ST segment	80–120 milliseconds
T-wave	160 milliseconds
QT interval	420 milliseconds or less if heart rate is 60 beats per minute (bpm)

APPENDIX 6

Effects of Various Drugs on ECG

Drug	ECG effect
Beta-blockers	Prolonged PR interval, decreases heart rate
Calcium channel blockers	Prolonged PR interval, decreased heart rate
Digoxin	Shortened QT interval, increased PR interval, decreased heart rate

Contd...

Contd...

Drug	ECG effect
Antiarrhythmics (Class I)	Widened QRS complex, prolonged QT interval
Antiarrhythmics (Class III)	Prolonged QT interval
Epinephrine	Increased heart rate, widened QRS complex
Atropine	Shortened PR interval, increased heart rate
Adenosine	Transient heart block, sinus bradycardia

APPENDIX 7

Tips for troubleshooting ECG equipment and obtaining accurate ECG readings:

- **Check the electrode placement:** Correct electrode placement is essential for accurate ECG readings. Make sure the electrodes are placed in the right locations, and that the skin is properly prepared.
- **Check the lead wires:** Ensure that the lead wires are in good condition and are not damaged. If they are damaged, replace them with new ones.
- **Check the power source:** If your ECG machine is not working, check if it is correctly plugged in and if the power source is working correctly.
- **Check the filters:** Check the filters in your ECG machine. If they are dirty or clogged, clean or replace them.
- **Perform calibration**: Perform calibration on your ECG machine. This will help ensure the accuracy of the readings.
- **Check the patient**: Sometimes the patient themselves can cause issues with ECG readings. Ensure the patient is calm and relaxed, not moving too much, and not wearing any jewelery or clothing that may interfere with the readings.

Index

Page numbers followed by *b* refer to box, *f* refer to figure, *fc* refer to flowchart, and *t* refer to table.

A

Acid-base
   disturbance 96
   imbalance 113
Acute coronary syndrome 78, 106
   complications of 86, 86*t*
   types of 78*f*
Acute myocardial infarction 68
   hallmarks of 82
   pattern of 83*f*
Acute pericarditis 7, 57, 121*f*
   pathognomonic of 57
Acute right ventricular dilatation 122
Acute sympathetic stress 68
Alcohol 70
Ambulatory electrocardiogram monitor 27
   type 27*b*
Amiodarone 107, 122
Amyloidosis 57, 60
Anasarca, evaluation of 171
Angina 86
Antiarrhythmic drugs 76, 117
Anticoagulant therapy 54
Athletes 111
Atrial activity, spontaneous 124
Atrial and ventricular
   pacing 124
   rate 118
   rhythm 56, 118
Atrial arrhythmia 86
Atrial depolarization 54
Atrial fibrillation 42, 42*f*, 89, 95, 95*f*, 96*f*, 111, 153, 154
   etiology of 96
   P waves 54
   treatment of 96, 97*fc*
   with pre-excitation 89
Atrial flutter 43, 43*f*, 89, 91, 92*f*
Atrial pacing 123
Atrial rate 43, 90, 92
Atrial rhythm 90, 92
Atrioventricular block 43, 55, 108
   causes for 111
   first degree 108, 109*f*
   lower-degree 57
   second degree 108, 109, 109*f*, 110*f*
   third degree 110, 110*f*
Atrioventricular nodal reentry tachycardia 148
Atrioventricular node 1, 5
   conduction 86, 111
   dysfunction 86
Augmented leads 23
Augmented limb leads 22, 24*f*

B

Bazett's formula 76, 76*f*
Beta-blockers 57, 107
   administration of 91
Biatrial enlargement 54
Biphasic deflection 17*f*
Bipolar leads 22, 23*f*
Bradyarrhythmias 107

Index

Bradycardia
    causes for 40*t*
    severe 115*f*
    tachycardia syndrome 111
Brugada syndrome 68, 158
Bundle branch 6*f*
    blocks 63, 72
    bundle of His and 1, 5, 54
    depolarization of 63

C

Caffeine 70
Calcium
    channel blockers 57, 91, 107
    disorders 118
Calculate intervals 37
Calculate rate 37
Caliper method 41*f*
Cardiac abnormality, specific 15
Cardiac aneurysm 68
Cardiac axis 45, 46
    thumb rule 49
Cardiac conduction system 1
Cardiac excitation, spread of 2
Cardiac failure 86
Cardiac rupture 86
Cardiac wall 86
Cardiogenic shock 86
Cardiomyopathy 57, 69, 96
Cardioversion 104
Catheter ablation 104
Cerebral hemorrhage 69
Cetirizine 122
Chagas disease 57
Chest
    discomfort 167
        clinical history of 78
    electrode 31
    leads 24
    pain
        central 146
        severe left-sided 165
Cholecystectomy 175
Chronic obstructive pulmonary disease 159
Citalopram 122
Clarithromycin 122
Classical method 45
Cocaine 70
Color codes 20*f*
Common cardiac arrhythmia 42
Conduction blocks 45
Conduction of impulses, rates of 4*t*
Cornell criteria 62
Coronary vasospasm 68
Cough, chronic 170

D

Defibrillation 104, 106
Depolarization
    vector of 45*f*
    waves of 17*f*
Depressions 157
Determine regularity 40
Dextrocardia 160
Digitalis 57, 70, 117
Digoxin effect 69, 120, 120*f*, 153
Diphtheria 57
Domperidone 122
Drugs 69
    and miscellaneous 120
    causing, list of 122
Dyspnea 170
    complains of 146
        acute 174
    worsening 159

E

Early repolarization 68
Ebstein's anomaly 54
Ectopics 72
Einthoven 11
    equilateral triangle 12*f*
Electrical impulse 45
Electrocardiogram 10, 42*f*, 43*f*, 44*f*, 89*f*, 101*f*, 107*f*, 109*f*, 113, 114*f*
    amplitude scale 13*f*

changes in 114*t*
characteristics 90, 92, 98, 100, 102, 103, 105
discovery of mechanism of 11
information on 27
interpret 177
manifestation 85
pacing in 123
strip 40*f*
technical aspects of 10
utility of 11
waveforms 6, 8*f*, 51
Electrocardiogram changes
acute pericarditis 121*f*
infarct 82
injury 79, 80*f*
ischemia 79, 80*f*
Electrocardiogram leads 13, 14*f*
correct placement of 27
Electrocardiogram paper
and timing 11
standard calibrations of 13*f*
Electrocardiographic tracings 78
Electrode placement 15, 31
Electrolyte 113
disturbance 96
imbalance 69, 76, 98, 106
severity of 113
Equiphasic approach 45
Erythromycin 122
Escitalopram 122
Ethanol abuse 69

F

Fatigue 162
Fexofenadine 122
Fibrillary waves 54, 95
First degree heart block 55, 55*f*
First-line pharmacologic therapy 105
Fluconazole 122

G

Gallbladder disease 70

H

Haloperidol 122
Heart
conduction system of 2*f*
natural pacemaker 123
rate, calculating 39*f*
rhythm, fast 44
wall of 84*f*
wiring system of 1
Heart block 108, 157
causes of 57*b*
complete 56, 110
third degree 56, 56*f*
Hernia surgery 166
Himalayan P waves 54
His bundle 109
Holter monitor 27, 28*f*
Hydroxyzine 122
Hypercalcemia 9, 118*f*
ECG features of 118
Hyperkalemia 57, 98, 114*f*, 115*f*
ECG 116*f*
features of 113
severe 115*f*, 161
Hypernatremia 113
Hypertension 96
Hypertrophic cardiomyopathy 68
Hypertrophy, assess for 37
Hyperventilation 69
Hypocalcemia 98
ECG features of 118
Hypokalemia 9, 70, 77, 98, 117*f*
ECG features of 117
severe 162
T inversion in 117*f*
Hypomagnesemia 98
Hyponatremia 113
Hypotension 147
Hypothermia 60, 68
Hypothyroid 60

I

Idioventricular rhythm 68, 99, 100*f*

Implantable cardioverter defibrillator 99, 104
Impulse
    conduction through heart 3f
    generation, rate of 5, 5t
    traveling away 82
Infarction, evidence of 37
Infiltrative diseases 57
Internodal atrial pathway 1
Internodal conduction pathways 4
Intracranial hemorrhage, setting of 77
Intraventricular extension 164
Irregular palpitations, history of 150
Ischemia 69, 76
Ischemic and nonspecific change 73f
Ischemic area 70f
Ischemic heart disease 96
    history of 149
Isoelectric segment 57

J

J point 66
J wave 7, 8, 9f
Jervell and Lange-Nielsen syndrome 77, 105
Junctional rhythm 89

L

Leads
    arrangement of 23, 26f
    twelve-possible 20f
Lead placement 23, 31, 34
    in special situations 16f
Lead reversal 29f
    electrocardiogram 29
Left anterior descending, causes of 48
Left atrial enlargement 53, 53f
Left axis deviation 47f
    causes of 48, 48b

Left bundle branch block 63, 64f, 64t, 65
Left leg, malleolus of 35
Left sternal edge 31
Left ventricular
    hypertrophy 62, 68, 169
        causes of 63t
    mural thrombus 86
    overload 70
Lenegre's disease 57
Lev's disease 57
Lidocaine 99
Limb
    electrode 34
    leads
        electrodes 20, 21f
        unipolar 22
Loop recorder 27

M

Magnesium sulfate 99
McGinn and White sign 122, 122f
Medical emergency 104
Medication 76
Metabolic acidosis 98, 106
Methadone 122
Midclavicular line 32
Mitral regurgitation 86
Mitral stenosis 96
Monomorphic ventricular tachycardia 102f
Multifocal atrial tachycardia 89
Myocardial infarction 69f, 78, 82, 111, 147
    electrocardiogram in 78
    localization of 82
Myocardial ischemia 70
Myocarditis 57, 60, 69, 70, 111
Myoglobin 78
Myxedema 72

N

Narrow complex tachydysrhythmias 89

Necrotic tissue 82
Non-ST elevation myocardial infarction 85
Non-ST segment elevation myocardial infarction 78
Normal axis deviation 47*f*

O

Ondansetron 122
Oxygen therapy 106

P

P wave 41, 52, 52*f*, 90
    abnormalities of 52, 52*f*, 54
    absent 54
    inverted 54
    loss of 115*f*
    polymorphic 54
Paced rhythm 68
Pacemaker 56, 123
    device 123
    type of 123
    ventricular 172
Pacing 72
Palpitations 98
Pancreatitis 70
Papillary muscle 86
Paroxysmal supraventricular tachycardia, mechanism of 94*f*
Pericardial disease 96
Pericardial effusion 60
Pericarditis 68, 69, 70, 86, 121, 121*f*
Peripheral embolus 86
Phenothiazines 76
Pheochromocytoma 70, 96
Pneumothorax 70
Polymorphic ventricular tachycardia 103*f*
Postcatheter ablation 111
Potassium
    chloride 99
    disorders 113
    high 68
    levels 114*t*
Potassium-to-sodium ratio 113
PR interval 54, 90
    short 57
PR segment 57, 58*f*
Precordial lead 18
    configurations 29*f*
    placement of 19*f*
    twelve-possible 19*f*
Pre-excitation syndromes 96
Premature ventricular complex 97, 98*f*
Pre-syncope, episode of 156
Prinzmetal's angina 68
Procainamide 57
Pulmonary embolism 68, 69, 70, 96, 121
Pulse disappears 106
Pulseless torsades 105
Purkinje cardiomyocytes 6
Purkinje fibers 6, 6*f*, 63
Purkinje system 1, 4
P-wave 107, 114, 118

Q

Q wave 58, 58*f*
    pathological 58, 59*f*
    prolongation 59*f*
QRS
    low voltage 60, 61*f*
    voltage, low 171
QRS axis 44
    determine 37
QRS complex 58, 66*f*, 90, 107, 114, 118
    high voltage 61
    measuring 60, 61*f*
    narrow 89
    shape of 45*f*
    variation in 60, 60*f*
    wide 63, 89
QT interval 7, 75, 76*f*, 114, 118
    calculation of 75
    long 77*f*, 117*f*

prolonged 75
short 75
QT prolongation 122
QT syndrome 75
  long 77
Quadrant approach 45, 46*f*
Quadriparesis 162
Quinidine 57, 117

R

Radiofrequency catheter ablation 99
Rapid ventricular response 95
Reciprocal changes 82, 84*f*
Recording electrocardiogram trace 35
Regular rhythm 54
Regurgitation 96
Restrictive cardiomyopathy 60
Reverse tick 120*f*
Rheumatic fever 57
Rhythm 40
  determine 37
  irregular 39
  irregularly irregular 95
Right atrial enlargement 52, 53*f*, 159
Right axis deviation 46*f*
  causes of 48, 48*b*
Right bundle branch block 63, 64*f*, 64*t*, 65, 66*f*, 121, 175
Right sternal edge 31
Right ventricular hypertrophy 61, 62*f*, 170
  causes of 63*t*
Risperidone 122
Road traffic accident 161
Romano-Ward syndrome 105
Rule of 300 37, 37*f*
  calculation of rate with 38*t*

S

S wave 59
  deep 62*f*

Salvador Dali sagging appearance 120
Sarcoidosis 57
Scleroderma 57
Second degree heart block 55, 55*f*, 56*f*
Sick sinus syndrome 111
Sickle cell disease 173
Sine wave 115*f*
Sinoatrial exit block 111
Sinoatrial node 123
  leads heart 4
  natural 123
  of Keith and Flack 4
Sinus
  arrest 111
  node dysfunction 86, 111, 112*f*
  P wave 123
  pause 42, 42*f*
  tachycardia 42, 42*f*, 89, 90, 90*f*, 91*f*, 121
Sinus arrhythmia 111
  loss of 91
Sinus bradycardia 41, 41*f*, 107, 107*f*, 111, 169, 176
  causes 107
  ECG characteristics 107
  medical management 107
Sinus rhythm 89, 89*f*
  normal 41, 41*f*
Smoker complains
  lightheadedness 152
  palpitations 152
Sokolow and Lyon criteria 63*f*
ST depression 67*f*
  causes of 72*f*
  reciprocal 121*f*
  types of 69*f*
ST elevation, significant 80, 80*b*, 81*f*
ST segment 7, 66, 67*f*
  depression 69, 82, 86*f*
  deviations 69*f*
ST segment elevation 68, 68*f*

Index

myocardial infarction 78
   presence of 82
Standard leads 23
Subarachnoid hemorrhage 69
Subendocardial ischemia 67, 67f
Subepicardial ischemia 67, 68f
Supraventricular tachycardia 44, 44f, 89, 93, 94f, 148
   paroxysmal 93
   with aberrancy 89
Sympathomimetics 96

T

T wave 68
   elevation and inversion 70f
   inversion 70, 72f
      deep 73, 73f
   morphology, types of 71f
   peaked 114f
   tall 73, 74f
Tachyarrhythmia 88, 88fc
Tachycardia
   causes for 40t
   ventricular 43, 43f, 89, 101, 101f
Tachydysrhythmia 88
Thumbs 49, 50
   left 49
Thyrotoxicosis 9, 96
Tissue 5
Torsades de pointes 44, 44f, 89, 104, 104f, 105
Tricyclic antidepressants 76
Troponin 78

U

U wave 7, 9, 77, 77f
   prominent 117f

Ulnar styloid process
   left arm 34
   right arm 34
Unconsciousness 106

V

Vagal tone, increased 111
Valvular heart disease 96
Variable block 89
Ventricular aneurysm 86
Ventricular arrhythmia 86
Ventricular enlargement 45
Ventricular escape rhythm 99
Ventricular fibrillation 43, 43f, 89, 105, 105f
Ventricular pacing 123
Ventricular rate 90, 92, 100
   controlled 96f
Ventricular repolarization 70f
Ventricular rhythm 90, 92
Ventricular septum 86
Voriconazole 122

W

Waveforms, formation of 16, 18f
Waves
   examine individual 37
   flutter 54
   formation of 17f
   genesis of 51f
Wenckebach phenomenon 108, 156
Wolff-Parkinson-White syndrome 57, 173

EU GSPR Authorised Reprsentative
Logos Europe, 9 rue Nicolas Poussin
1700, La Rochelle, France
Phone: +33 (0) 6 67 93 73 78
E-mail: contact@logoseurope.eu

www.ingramcontent.com/pod-product-compliance
Ingram Content Group UK Ltd.
Pitfield, Milton Keynes, MK11 3LW, UK
UKHW021146270226
468476UK00001B/2